# The Wellness Ethic

# The Wellness Ethic

How to **Thrive** in an Unpredictable World
(Where Stupid Things Can Happen)

## Mark Reinisch

Seneca
House

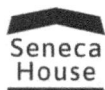

Seneca
House

Published by Seneca House Press, Charleston, South Carolina

The information in this book was derived from extensive research by the author, consultation with experts, and insights from personal experiences. The methods and practices depicted have not been customized for individual needs, and the author, though he has been diligent in preparing this book, makes no warranties regarding the accuracy or completeness of the concepts portrayed. Therefore, readers are urged to consult with appropriate professionals, such as doctors, financial advisors, and other licensed practitioners, before trying out anything consequential depicted in this book. The author assumes no responsibility or liability for any injuries or damages that could result from practicing concepts contained within *The Wellness Ethic*.

This book was written by a human being (not artificial intelligence).

For information about this title, contact the publisher:

Seneca House Press
Charleston, South Carolina
SenecaHousePress.com
SenecaHousePress@gmail.com

Printed in the United States of America

First Edition

Trademarks: Nurture the Wonderful Gift of Your Existence®, Self-Actualized Genius®, and Wellness Ethic®

Illustrations: Danny Burgess
Editors: Nancy Pile, Stuart Horwitz, Emma Reinisch
Cover Design: 1106 Design, Mark Reinisch
Interior Design: 1106 Design, Mark Reinisch

Library of Congress Control Number: 2025909416

ISBNs:
979-8-9916049-1-8 (hardcover)
979-8-9916049-0-1 (softcover)
979-8-9916049-2-5 (eBook)

*To my beautiful and caring wife, Kristen,*
*who has brought love, meaning, and joy to my life.*

*To my brilliant and adventurous children,*
*Audrey and Emma, who have taught me more about*
*living than a thousand books could ever teach.*

*To my parents, who helped me build a solid*
*foundation to support a lifetime of dreams.*

*To my brother, Bob, who motivated me to strive*
*beyond my years as only an annoying older sibling could.*

*To my friends, who have kept life interesting*
*by providing endless comedic fodder.*

*To the inspirational teachers I've had in my life—some*
*I have been blessed to know personally; others I've known*
*through history and literature—who guided me to find my life*
*purpose and live it with passion, confidence, and resilience.*

# Background Stuff

## Definitions

**Self-Actualized Genius (SAGe)**

*noun*

1. a person who has an exceptional ability to realize wellness—to the extent they can influence—by bringing their best self forward
2. a person's internal guiding force that encourages them to prioritize wellness in their life

**wellness**

*noun*

the state of being healthy in mind, body, and spirit, especially as an outcome of intentional pursuit

**Wellness Ethic**

*noun*

a value-centered devotion to wellness and its intrinsic ability to better one's existence and society at large

**Wellness Ethic journey**

*noun*

a wellness-centered progression in life that a person intentionally forges to generate love

# A Bit More on Being
# a Self-Actualized Genius (SAGe)

According to the American psychologist Abraham Maslow's hierarchy of needs theory, people are motivated by five needs: (1) physiological necessities (food, water, shelter), (2) safety, (3) love and belonging, (4) esteem, and (5) self-actualization, the highest state. A self-actualized person realizes their full potential in life. As Maslow wrote in 1943 (please excuse his antiquated masculine prose): "A musician must make music, an artist must paint, a poet must write, if he is to be ultimately happy. What a man *can* be, he *must* be."[1]

To expand upon this concept, a self-actualized person—or **Self-Actualized Genius (SAGe)** in Wellness Ethic-speak—prioritizes thriving in their life. Wellness, to the extent that it can be influenced, is the natural outcome.

**Your SAGe represents your best self.** It is your internal guiding force that nudges you to promote well-being. When your SAGe steers your life, you:

- know your life purpose and move forward in that direction with passion, confidence, and resilience.

- tend to your mental, physical, and spiritual well-being.

- feel connected to the universe and develop loving relationships.

- have a positive, value-centered approach to life that honors your autonomy and authenticity.

- choose love-centered responses to your circumstances.

- pursue experiences that bring love, happiness, and fulfillment to your life and the lives of others.

- minimize suffering because you understand that impermanence is an inescapable reality of how the universe works.

- accept the perfection of your imperfect existence.

*The Wellness Ethic* will guide you in activating your Self-Actualized Genius to boost your wellness so you can thrive in an unpredictable world (where stupid things can happen).

## The 80/20 Rule

Thousands of books on wellness topics have been written throughout the ages, and if you tried to adopt all their practices, you would need a thousand lifetimes. There's a better way to improve your wellness—applying the 80/20 rule—and you can do it in your lifetime.

The 80/20 rule, also known as the Pareto principle, was derived from the work of Italian economist Vilfredo Pareto. It states that approximately 80% of the results (outcomes) are driven by 20% of the actions (inputs).

When you apply the 80/20 rule to your life, it can be a game changer. For example, the 80/20 rule suggests that 80% of the benefits of spirituality can be attained by embracing just a few essential tenets, the most vital 20% of spiritual practices. Similarly, 80% of the benefits of taking care of your body can be realized by simply adopting the most vital 20% of physical wellness practices. The 80/20 rule encourages you to keep it simple by focusing your valuable time and energy on what's most impactful (also known as "the vital few").

**In *The Wellness Ethic*, I'll apply the 80/20 rule to uncover the essence of wellness topics—the handful of concepts and practices that offer the most value to the average person—and will avoid covering every nuance.** This approach will make wellness accessible and actionable. We won't let perfect be the enemy of good.

Just so you know, my alternative to taking the 80/20 approach would have been to author a 12,000-page treatise covering every imaginable facet of wellness. I seriously considered doing that because I have a lot of time on my hands, but then I stumbled upon the cautionary tale of Madeleine de Scudéry. In the seventeenth century, de Scudéry wrote *Artamène ou le Grand Cyrus*, a bloated, 13,095-page romance novel that was a stern test of endurance and kept readers away from tending to basic life necessities, like eating, plowing fields, and going to the outhouse.

I aspire to avoid a similar fate with *The Wellness Ethic* and will apply the 80/20 rule to keep it under 2,500 pages (to be safe).

You're welcome.

## A Quote from Mr. Thoreau

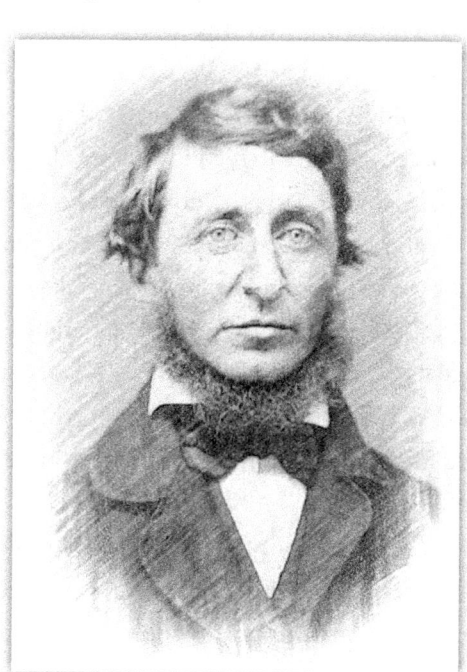

*I learned this, at least, by my experiment: that if one advances confidently in the direction of his dreams, and endeavors to live the life which he has imagined, he will meet with a success unexpected in common hours.*

—Henry David Thoreau, American naturalist and philosopher

# Contents

# Introduction

Step a little closer and imagine your mind, body, and spirit as a dance troupe swinging and spinning to the beat of your life purpose. Would that harmony saturate your life with love and help you thrive? Does feeling and sharing love represent the meaning of life, the ultimate aim of your existence? The short answer to those questions is a resounding *hell yes!*

But life is unpredictable. It's a potpourri of triumphs and struggles, with good fortune that bounces your way as if guided by Divinity, and stupid things thrown in your path by Chance. It's easy to fall into the habit of impulsively *reacting* to your circumstances, often with mixed results, rather than *responding* with your best self—your Self-Actualized Genius (SAGe)—to bring love into your life.

Being intentional with your response to life's unpredictable offerings is essential to your well-being because, no matter how hard you try, **you can't tame life—you can only tame your response to life**.

Mastering that universal truth has been a lifelong pursuit of mine.

## This Crazy Little Thing Called My Life

I'll be vulnerable throughout this book, and now is one of those times. Before the Wellness Ethic, I struggled with life and how to live it. I obsessed over my perceived flaws and unfulfilled dreams. Whatever joy I experienced

1

always had an asterisk next to it—I knew it was just a matter of time before my all-consuming "troubles" would crowd out the good feeling.

You see, I was aware for decades that I was blowing it. But I didn't sit back idly. Every year, I had oodles of conviction when I launched my New Year's resolutions to fix my life. Unfortunately, that resolve was a fickle companion. Life would soon interfere with my best-laid plans, and my transformation to "Mark Reinisch 2.0" would fizzle.

Then, in 2018, I had the epiphany of epiphanies that promised to serve as the catalyst for the lasting change I ached for. It was a eureka moment that didn't quite compel me to run through the streets in the buff like Archimedes after discovering the law of buoyancy—public decency statutes have evolved over the last two millennia—but, for me, it was a big deal.

My breakthrough idea was to write a book about wellness and apply the wisdom to my life to become happier and more fulfilled. If I could learn how to eclipse the blinding daylight between inspired living and my actual existence, I knew I could help others do the same.

I only saw the upside of committing to this mission. To start with, I was confident the experience would get me closer to realizing my best self. That excited me. Moreover, I would create a legacy for my children. Long after I was gone, they would have a book they could turn to whenever they wanted to tap into the wisdom I had accumulated in my life. That comforted me.

As far as achieving traditional literary success, as measured by royalties and bestseller lists, that's not what this was about. Even if the book were self-published, with fewer than ten copies sold (bought by guilt-ridden friends and family members, no doubt), I would have a book on my book-shelf written by me! It would become an exclamation point in my life—a life that didn't need punctuation, but something inside of me felt otherwise.

To launch writing *The Wellness Ethic*, I wanted to start by baselining how I perceived my life before adopting the wellness principles I would soon uncover. With that intention, on October 20, 2018, I documented my pre-Wellness Ethic mindset.

As you'll see by the rantings that quickly consumed my narrative, I had a heaping helping of issues to work through. Before the Wellness Ethic, I was the poster child for the *glass-is-half-empty* mindset. In fact, not only did I see the glass as half-empty, but I also felt like the glass had a leak in it to boot!

## My Pre-Wellness Ethic Mindset—October 20, 2018

My life is quite good, actually. Don't worry. I just knocked on wood and obliterated all the jinxing forces unleashed when I made that bold pronouncement.

I know my blessings are many. I have a loving marriage—my wife and I celebrated our twenty-fifth wedding anniversary this year! My two daughters are forces of nature—spirited, wildly talented, and compassionate. I'm healthy (*knock, knock, knock*). I've had a successful career in corporate America.

I've also pursued side hustles that have kept life interesting over the years, including launching a social media start-up, writing a dozen comedic screenplays, and running a part-time life coaching business. Some ventures didn't go as far as my lofty ambitions, while others got decent traction.

When I add it all up, my life has been good by any reasonable standard. So, why the hell am I not happy?!

I'll tell you why! Let's start with my job. A few months ago, I got a big promotion. Cool, huh? But I didn't get a raise, stock options, a better corporate title, or even a $5 Arby's gift card for the privilege of taking on vast new responsibilities and assuming significant career risk. Argh!

I'll now toggle over to one of my side hustles: launching a social media platform with a co-founder and team. We sold the business for restricted stock options last December. That should be a cause for celebration! Not so fast. After we closed the deal, I was bilked out of $7,000 by someone involved in the transaction. To make matters worse, the company that acquired our business had planned to work with our team to launch a 2nd Gen version of our platform, but the post-sale partnership never got off the ground. My negative self-talk about these setbacks has become a deafening earworm!

Then I get to my personal life. I want to experience the outdoors with my family in grand ways. I want to rekindle my passion for screenwriting. I want to travel to enchanting lands steeped in art, history, savory cuisine, and architectural wonders. I would love to learn how to paint.

But I work fifty-five to sixty hours a week, sometimes more. My Monday through Friday commute lasts an hour *each way*. I get home around 7:00 p.m., have dinner, connect with my family for thirty minutes or so, shower, and then climb into bed, beaten to a pulp. Rinse and repeat, rinse and repeat, day after day after monotonous day.

My weekends aren't better. Work has gobbled up my weekends like a pack of rabid raccoons having a feeding frenzy at an all-you-can-eat buffet. Sadly, corporate America has become the dominatrix in my life (absent the sex, for the record, in case you had doubts). And now, just to make life more interesting, I think my employer is about to be acquired. So much for job security!

My harsh reality is that I'm witnessing a life I'm not living. I've been glued to the passenger seat of a speeding car, zipping through life, watching happiness pass by in a blur. I've been alive for 18,155 days, and I still haven't figured out how to slow down and nurture the wonderful gift of my existence.

**Nurture the wonderful gift of my existence.** That needs to become the tagline of my life. It's my only real need; everything else is a want. Hmm.

I have so much opportunity for growth. But I'm thrilled that I'm taming my response to that opportunity by writing this book and going on a Wellness Ethic journey. My mission may prove to be hard, but unhappiness is harder.

## Foreshadowings—What to Expect from *The Wellness Ethic* Experience

My guess is you're reading this book because, like me, you want more out of your life—more joy, calm, purpose, health, more of something that has been stubbornly elusive. Or perhaps you know the author and realize that the only way he'll stop bugging you is if you just suck it up and read his book. Whatever your motivation, I'm glad you're here. I wrote *The Wellness Ethic* to make wellness accessible and actionable to help people supercharge their lives.

*The Wellness Ethic* is divided into twelve sections, with each section covering a different wellness topic. Most sections contain two chapters: a "story" chapter followed by a "wellness" chapter. Both chapters work together to bring the wellness topics to life.

Story chapters depict experiences from my life that I put through the Wellness Ethic lens. They set up the concepts covered in the wellness chapters by providing real examples of what good and not-so-good look like.

Wellness chapters utilize the 80/20 rule (80% of the results come from 20% of the most impactful actions) to teach the essence of wellness topics, including mind, body, spirit, relationships, adopting change, and others. At the end of the wellness chapters, I incorporated simple exercises to help you decide how to move forward with what you've learned. I also completed them, so you'll see how I approached my own Wellness Ethic journey.

As you read *The Wellness Ethic*, taking action on what you learn will be essential to realizing the best version of yourself (your SAGe). Otherwise, as instructors will tell you after a class: *If you don't use it, you'll lose it.* With that in mind, I'll offer suggestions on how you can get the most out of this book:

○ *Have a bias for action.* Without action, you're just engaging in wishful thinking. As you move forward, embrace experimentation. You may fall short at times—it happens to all of us—but you'll also find plenty of ideas that will work. One thing is sure: Time marches on whether you choose to nurture the wonderful gift of your existence or not.

○ *Start small to get quick wins.* Focus on adopting smaller and easier changes in your life to build your change-adoption muscles (and your confidence). Then, expand to more challenging intentions.

○ *Experience "The Wellness Ethic" with friends.* Form a group and progress through this book together. Meet regularly to discuss the chapters and what you're doing to move forward. Share ideas. Celebrate wins. Support one another during challenging times. Besides helping with motivation, the camaraderie will make your Wellness Ethic journey more enjoyable.

○ *Explore topics further.* Books, classes, podcasts, experts, the internet—embrace learning! You can also visit WellnessEthic.com to access my wellness blog and sign up for my *Sunday SAGe* newsletter.

**Above all else, have fun!** Have fun reading *The Wellness Ethic* (I had fun writing it). Have fun putting the concepts into practice.

Self-improvement shouldn't be a burden. Sure, sometimes you'll feel frustrated when you face obstacles. But struggle breeds wisdom, and you can use that wisdom to break through with the growth you seek. As you move forward, you'll soon find that adopting change gets easier and easier once you experience the energizing good that comes your way.

Let's begin our Wellness Ethic journey!

○   ○   ○

# Enter the Wellness Ethic

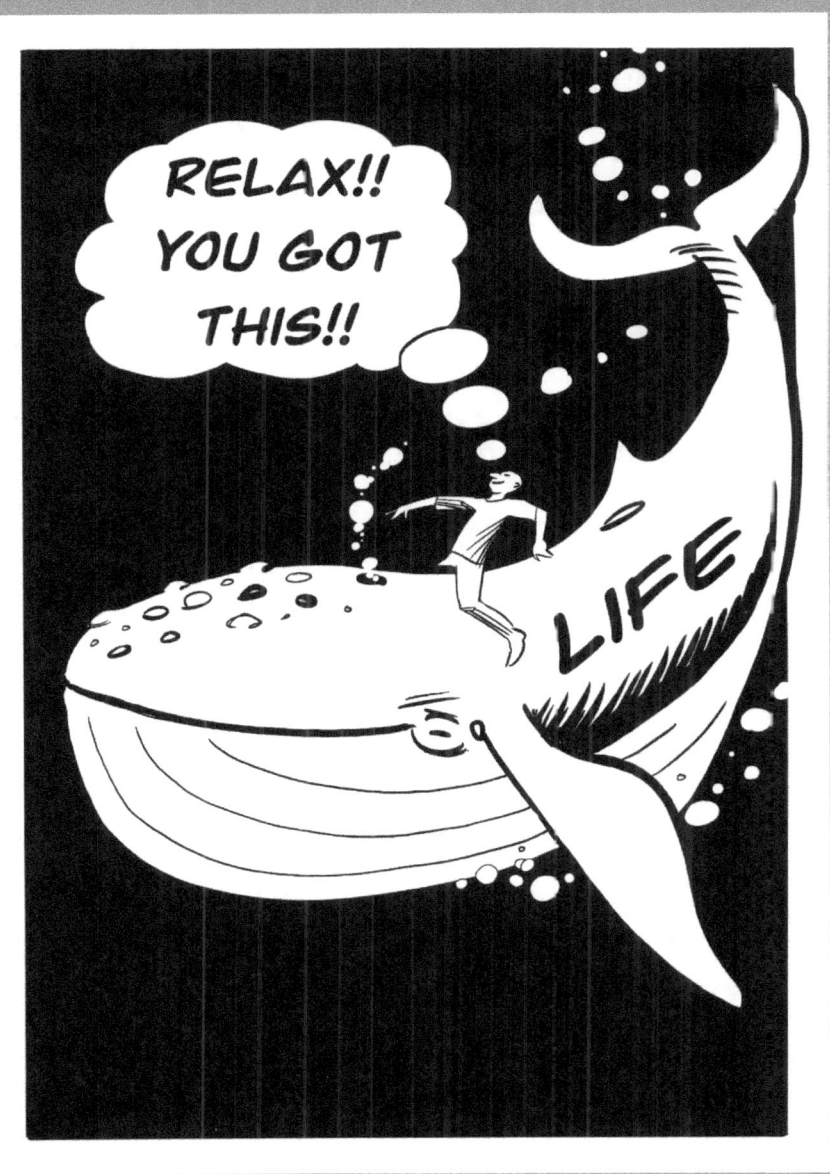

# CHAPTER 1

# A Story of Beginning

When I entered the bustling Charlotte airport to board a plane to Chicago, two weighty thoughts ricocheted in my brain: *I'm not sure if my life is worth living*, and *Gosh dangit, I better have an aisle seat!*

I certainly had no clue that this Bank of America business trip taken over fifteen years ago would shake up my life. Why would it? I had traveled at least a hundred times in my career, and the routine was as predictable as the regret you feel after eating an entire box of Girl Scout cookies in one sitting.

At the destination, I would work like a sled dog into the night. I'd then settle in at the hotel and watch cable news as I mindlessly ate room service a grade above a freezer-burned TV dinner. After that, I would surrender to a restless night of sleep. When my trip's mission was done, I'd drag my weary spirit home. Business trips were just another example of being suffocated in a common-law marriage to my squandered existence. Sorry for the mainline of gloom, but that was my afflicted mindset at the time.

As I stood in the Charlotte airport check-in line, waiting for my final seat assignment, my anxiety levels were elevated—I must have an aisle seat! I will book well in advance to ensure I get one. But sometimes the airline switches planes before departure and reassigns me to a middle or window seat. I believe this happens because, in the past, I once answered "both" when a flight attendant asked me to choose between pretzels and Biscoff cookies. This transgression clearly offended the Greek God of Airline Snacks, and I've been cursed ever since.

Why is an aisle seat so important? I'm six-foot-three and claustrophobic, so maximum stretch-out space is imperative. *The Incident* also plays an outsized role in my neurosis. I probably should elaborate, but be forewarned that this will be heart-wrenching.

Early in my career, I was sitting in a window seat as my direct, five-hour flight from Charlotte to Seattle was boarding at the pace of a drunken sloth. The air conditioning was off, I was sweating, and my legs were restless, so I started to obsess over my growing discomfort.

Then, as I stretched my irritable legs under the seat in front of me, my row filled with grown men—the walls were closing in! I knew there was no conceivable way I could cope with a long flight when I felt like the bottom fish in a can of anchovies. I most certainly couldn't ask someone with an aisle seat to switch seats with me. Yeah, right. That would be like being lost and asking for directions. Why would anyone in their right mind behave so irrationally?

I had no choice but to get the professionals involved. I navigated to the front of the boarding plane, squeezing past annoyed passengers, to discuss my sad plight with the flight attendant. She confirmed the flight was full, and I had no options unless I asked someone to switch seats with me. I politely explained that the probability of that happening was zero, so I needed to book another flight. Problem solved, right? Nope. Not even close.

What I didn't count on, not in any of my prior calculations on how this dire situation could possibly end, was that the wily flight attendant would have a customer service moment for the ages. As I stood in the aisle near the front of the plane, she went on the plane's loudspeaker and offered a bottle of wine to anyone who would give up their aisle seat for my window seat. Everyone stared at me, the sorry, pitiful schmuck who was too much of a helpless little baby to simply ask someone sitting by him if they would switch seats!

But her Hail Mary scheme worked. After a few minutes, someone in the back of the plane struck the deal.

As I embarked upon my walk of shame to my new seat, the flight attendant, clearly in cahoots with my old nemesis, the Greek God of Airline Snacks, decided to take my humiliation up a notch. She announced to the passengers that a kind traveler had accepted the deal, which promptly drew everyone's attention back to me! The passengers applauded as they stared at my beet-red face. Air travel became the bane of my existence after that mortifying experience.

I'm glad I got that off my chest. It was cathartic. Now back to the Chicago trip. Thankfully, check-in was successful—aisle seat secured! I then boarded the plane. As I sat in my cramped seat, I had a thought. It wasn't the first time such a thought had entered my mind while waiting on a runway—it was an acknowledgment of how I viewed my life. I thought if the plane crashed and everyone survived but me, I would be okay with that.

In the big picture, I had a lot to live for. I loved my family. I was healthy. I had a good job. I was pursuing my screenwriting dreams. But I was also in a decades-long state of despair. Every vision I had for my life that wasn't manifesting in my reality blotted out the positive. The issues I was dealing with accounted for 5% to 10% of my existence, which was a mere nit in the grand scheme. But when someone feels hopeless, perspective is lost, the good gets eclipsed by the bad, and the small part of your life that isn't going well can feel like your entire world.

I arrived in Chicago and checked into my hotel room. I ate dinner as I channel-surfed, and soon stumbled upon a PBS special featuring Dr. Wayne Dyer discussing his book *Change Your Thoughts—Change Your Life: Living the Wisdom of the Tao*. In the book, Dyer wrote a chapter for each of the eighty-one verses of the *Tao Te Ching*, the 2,500-year-old spiritual text by Lao-Tzu that serves as the foundation for Taoism. I was intrigued enough by what I heard that I went to bed thinking I needed to remember to buy Dyer's book.

After a few days of work, I was ready to head home. I took a taxi to the airport, checked in for my flight, and then bought the book at a store.

Once I got situated at my gate, I started reading. It was like I was struck by a superbolt of lightning thrown directly from the hand of Zeus!

I was blown away when I read Dyer's Taoist-inspired words: "Don't try so hard to make something work—simply allow." That was radically different from how I approached my life. I loved his perspective that "there is no way to happiness; rather, happiness is the way." But it was his following passage that convinced me there was no going back to my old way of thinking:

> *. . . Imagine yourself as an otter just living your "otterness." You're not good or bad, beautiful or ugly, a hard worker or a slacker . . . you're simply an otter, moving through the water or on the land freely, peacefully, playfully, and without judgments.*[1]

I closed the book after forty pages to gather my astounded senses. How could I try to force outcomes out of my control, like I had been doing for years, when I now understood that it creates friction with the natural way life flows? Why should I judge myself harshly when I was exactly like the universe intended me to be? Why should I search in vain for happiness when happiness was already inside of me in abundance, just waiting to be tapped into? I realized I was empowered to choose happiness over despair. For me, this was a revolutionary way to approach life.

I knew I had to surrender to the call and act upon this profound wisdom. There wasn't a choice. It was like I was awakened from a deep sleep by a bonk on the head from a waterlogged two-by-four!

> *When the student is ready, the teacher will appear.*
> —Lao-Tzu

A few months later, while traveling on business, I had another life-altering experience. This time, it came from a most unlikely source: an American Express ad featuring Larry David that I saw in an airline magazine.

David, the creator of *Curb Your Enthusiasm* and co-creator of *Seinfeld*, is a comedic legend. The ad was a funny profile that detailed his "Proudest accomplishment," favorite "In-flight movie," and others. One of the topics was "Occupation," which he listed as "Life Coach." I found it amusing and moved on.

But the idea of pursuing a career as a life coach tugged at me over the ensuing weeks. Why not become a life coach? I loved helping people. My corporate background was in continuous improvement and change adoption. I could be a good coach. So I signed up for a yearlong life coaching certification program through the International Coach Academy.

The life coaching certification experience was intensive as I progressed through the requirements with my fellow students and built a part-time coaching business in parallel. Launching a business was exciting, but I was most energized by the personal transformation I was experiencing.

As part of the training, I was introduced to lifestyle design and applied the concepts to my life. I started a daily exercise regimen, which I've continued to this day. I improved my diet. I began to do yoga. I carved out time each week to read books on spirituality and how the mind works. All those changes, big and small, had a cumulative effect on my well-being. And to my delight, my positive outlook improved with every step forward.

When I look back at that time, well over a decade ago, I now have the wisdom to realize that my life coaching journey wasn't really about starting a business. That made life interesting for a while, but it wasn't why I went down that path. Being trained as a life coach—and acting upon what I learned—was the key to breaking out of my cycle of despair. The mindset transformation I experienced saved my life in many ways.

But I have also learned over the years that you must continuously nurture your well-being, or it can slowly decline. Although I am light-years beyond where I was during my darkest days, as you can tell from reading the introduction to this book, I am nowhere near where I need to be. That will change, however—I'm on a Wellness Ethic journey to nurture the wonderful gift of my existence. That awareness alone has already created positive energy in my life, and it will only get better.

Before we move on to the next chapter, I'd like to tie up a few loose ends concerning air travel. Did I mention that airlines charge for everything? What's next? Charging convenience fees to use the lavatory? Then there's the serious issue of premium boarding groups. Why are there so many? Platinum Elite, Executive Platinum, Platinum Pro, Junior Executive Platinum—I've accepted that I can't get into any of them, but I don't like being confused! We need a congressional hearing on this. And don't get me started about people who recline their seats when someone tall is sitting behind them. Oh, the outrage! All right, all right, I'm getting worked up.

Let me try to calm my mind by putting air travel through the Wellness Ethic lens. If it weren't for air travel, I probably wouldn't have become a life coach, and who knows if my mindset would have improved? Airlines have allowed me to travel on business and partner with talented colleagues. I've visited my children. I've gone on family vacations throughout the United States and parts of Europe, connecting with diverse cultures and experiencing awe and wonder. When I add it up, that's a lot of happiness that has been brought into my life.

After thinking more about it, I'll choose to have a positive mindset about air travel rather than dwelling on the 5% to 10% I don't like. I'll focus on what makes me happy.

o   o   o

# CHAPTER 2

# For the Love of Wellness Models

At the beginning of this book, I defined "Wellness Ethic" as *a value-centered devotion to wellness and its intrinsic ability to better one's existence and society at large.* Does that definition make your brain hurt? Imagine how I felt when I wrote it! I know it can seem complicated, but it really isn't. Having a Wellness Ethic means you're committed to wellness because you know that it improves your life and makes the world better.

When you're devoted to wellness, you empower the best version of yourself—your Self-Actualized Genius (SAGe)—to guide your life so you can thrive. If I created a word cloud to describe that flourishing state (I like you, so I won't), you would see words like *positivity, love, purpose, calm, satisfying experiences, health, joy, character, acceptance, fulfillment, relationships, mindfulness,* and *gratitude.*

Though it may be less obvious, society also benefits from your wellness because a "well" person lifts the lives of others. This can be done in small ways, like a kind interaction with a store clerk that brightens their day, or in significant ways, such as volunteering at a nonprofit or raising a compassionate child. When you're well, you share your time, talents, and love with others so they can thrive.

Thriving in an unpredictable world (where stupid things can happen) requires you to design—and live—your life in a way that promotes wellness. Lifestyle design is integral to the Wellness Ethic, so we'll explore it further.

# Lifestyle Design—A Quick Primer

Lifestyle design is a topic that has generated a lot of attention post-pandemic, with companies and employees debating the impact remote, hybrid, and in-office work has on happiness and productivity. The premise of lifestyle design is to intentionally mold your life into an everyday existence that satisfies you. The desired outcome is well-being. Lifestyle design includes what you do—personally and professionally—where you do it, how much time you spend doing it, and with whom. It covers maintaining your life, such as managing money, and how you tend to mind, body, and spirit.

With lifestyle design, the objective is to get to the heart of what you *really* want in life and then make it your reality. Lifestyle design inspires you to open your mind to possibilities. It also requires trade-offs. Consider these scenarios:

- A single mother who works in the tech sector is unfulfilled but needs her job to pay the bills and support her teenage son. She would love to attend culinary school to become a chef.

- A college graduate wants to travel the world for a year but feels pressure to start his teaching career. He has college loans to pay off and is in a two-year relationship with someone who could be "the one."

- A remarkably delightful guy in his early thirties has a house in Ohio and a young family. He recently received a job promotion. But his passion is filmmaking, and he just won a full scholarship to a film school in British Columbia (a real scenario from my life decades ago).

How would you move forward if you were in their shoes? How would a life partner factor into the equation? What difficult choices and compromises would you make, and what would be the impact on your well-being? Imagine choosing a path without being in touch with your values and life purpose. It would be like playing a game of blindfolded dodgeball. Good luck with that!

Or imagine choosing the path of least resistance without trying to find a creative way to move forward with your dreams. You would be scooting over from the driver's seat in your life to the passenger's seat. Would you be fully satisfied? Would you always wonder, "What if?"

These examples illustrate why lifestyle design is essential to your well-being. When you design your life to promote wellness, you live on your terms to the extent you can control. You find the right combination of personal and professional pursuits that align with your life purpose and make you happy. You cultivate loving relationships. You strengthen your mind, body, and spirit to provide positive energy to engage in life. You learn the value of saying "no" to opportunities so you can say "yes" to things that matter more. Lifestyle design isn't a one-and-done process. It requires tuning as life happens. It involves short- and long-term thinking. Lifestyle design is an art and a science.

## You Have Already Designed Your Life! Congratulations?

Whether you realize it or not, you have already designed your life. You have chosen how you make ends meet, which interests you explore, and how you care for your body. You have decided where you live, whom you have relationships with, and which dreams you pursue (or have long since forgotten). How is your lifestyle design working for you? Are congratulations in order?

If you have aligned your world with what satisfies you, you're probably getting the most out of your life (or close to it). Perhaps you've even inhaled the rarefied air of a self-actualized existence. If your approach to life has been unintentional, your satisfaction is likely uneven, with some days better than others. But no matter where you're at, three things hold true:

O *You can't change the past.* So don't beat yourself up over past mistakes or missed opportunities. They're in your wake. Learn what you can, make amends if necessary, and move on.

○ *You want to be satisfied today.* So be intentional with how you live your life. Promote wellness in all that you do. It's the key to thriving.

○ *You want a satisfying tomorrow.* So control what you can control and put yourself in the best position for a happy and fulfilling future.

Focusing on wellness is the best way to position yourself for a satisfying today and tomorrow. This brings us to the Wellness Ethic.

## The Wellness Ethic Lifestyle Design

The Wellness Ethic has seven core components: *mind, body, spirit, relationships, personal pursuits, professional pursuits,* and *lifestyle maintenance.* When these aspects of your life work together harmoniously and are all guided by *love,* your life hits its stride—you thrive. Here is a model to illustrate:

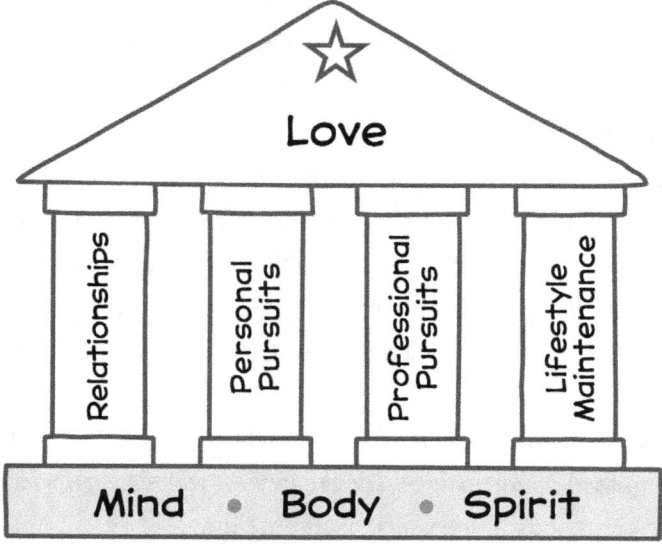

## Love

Designing your life should always start with one fundamental question: *What is the desired outcome of your life?* The answer to that question becomes your North Star, your compass, which guides you in how to live your life and what company to keep—practically all aspects of your life should align with your North Star. The Wellness Ethic believes that *feeling and sharing love*—the meaning of life—would be an excellent choice to serve as your North Star.

Love is a warm, emotional feeling of affection, care, and connection toward someone or something. When you feel and share love, you feel alive. You are happiest and most fulfilled when you love yourself, love what you're doing, love the person you're with, and love the positive impact you have in the world.

Love is everything. Think about how you feel when you go on a date with someone you love. Or when you do a good deed, care for someone, or accomplish something meaningful. Love is what we live for. It is the desired outcome of our lives. In fact, I'd suggest that our life success is a function of our wellness and the love we create *to the extent we can control*. Here's the equation:

## Life Success = Feeling Love + Sharing Love = Wellness

The rest of this book will focus on wellness as the catalyst to manifest love in our lives and within others. **Love is the Wellness Ethic's North Star.**

## The Foundation

A healthy mind, body, and spirit foundation generates positive energy that fuels your Wellness Ethic journey. That energy comes from the love you feel, an upbeat mindset, serenity, physical vitality, higher purpose, and your SAGe's all-knowing wisdom. A sturdy foundation supports a satisfying life.

*Your mind*—and the emotions and perceptions it creates—influences your happiness. When you're happy, you feel love toward the moment.

*Your body* provides the means for you to engage in life. When you care for your body, you live longer and have the energy to do what satisfies you.

*Your spirit* is your life force, the nonphysical essence of you. It represents your life purpose, humanity, values, and loving connection to others. When the way you live your life aligns with your spirit, you feel like you're a part of something greater than yourself. You develop a fulfilling sense of satisfaction, knowing your time on earth is well spent.

All three—mind, body, and spirit—are interconnected. For example, prolonged mental stress can lead to cardiovascular issues. When you exercise, your brain releases hormones (endorphins) that improve your mood. Practicing mindfulness helps you feel a deeper connection between yourself and the universe, which fosters spiritual well-being.

## The Pillars

The pillars of the Wellness Ethic—relationships, personal pursuits, professional pursuits, and lifestyle maintenance—are your SAGe's playground to manifest love.

- ○ *Relationships*: Our life satisfaction is influenced by how we connect with life partners, friends, family, colleagues, acquaintances, and even pets (of course pets are included—I dare you to tell them they're not!).

- ○ *Personal Pursuits*: These pursuits engage you in life and round out your existence. They include activities you choose to spend your free time pursuing, such as hobbies, traveling, sports, and reading.

- ○ *Professional Pursuits*: How you earn a living significantly impacts your satisfaction. When your job aligns with your life purpose, you're engaged in your work. When it's not, it can feel like a chore.

○ *Lifestyle Maintenance*: These activities help your life function. They include money management, housework, shopping, and others.

The foundation and the pillars are the essence of the Wellness Ethic. I recognize that you may feel overwhelmed. But don't worry. We'll keep it simple by utilizing the 80/20 rule to focus on what matters most. And you'll decide the pace of your Wellness Ethic journey. You may choose to travel with a sense of urgency or at a more measured stride. You'll know what works for you.

Here's another reason not to worry: I've devoted chapters 3 through 6 to building life skills that will help you gain traction with improving your wellness. You'll learn how to choose your SAGe-inspired response to the opportunities in your life to position for the best outcomes. You'll also discover ways to build habits and adopt changes that make wellness attainable *and* sustainable. So before we drill into the details of the Wellness Ethic model—starting with spirituality in chapter 7 (it'll provide purpose for your journey)—you'll be equipped with valuable insights and skills to help you translate what you learn in this book into actions that move your life forward.

At this point, I'd be remiss if I didn't remind you of what a wise person once said about self-improvement: "**Above all else, have fun!**" With that spirit in mind, let's advance confidently in the direction of our dreams!

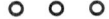

## Move Forward on Your Wellness Ethic Journey!

(1) Fill in the chart to create a wellness baseline of where you are today versus where you would like to be in a year. (Note: My example follows.)

Current State: *Rate how you are doing with each Wellness Ethic component. Use a scale of 1 to 10, with 1 = "I'm performing abysmally" and 10 = "I'm thriving."*

Ideal State: *Rate where you would like to be in a year using the same scale as the Current State.*

Gap: *Gap = Current score minus Ideal score. If the gap is negative, there's room for improvement. Circle your top priorities.*

| Wellness Ethic | Current | Ideal | Gap |
|---|---|---|---|
| Love | | | |
| Mind | | | |
| Body | | | |
| Spirit | | | |
| Relationships | | | |
| Personal Pursuits | | | |
| Professional Pursuits | | | |
| Lifestyle Maintenance | | | |
| Observations | | | |
| | | | |

(2) Advanced Topics (going beyond the 80/20): Research "Mediterranean lifestyle" and "Scandinavian lifestyle" on the internet to see if there are practices you want to incorporate into your life. Studies have shown that both lifestyle designs can produce significant (and exciting) wellness benefits.

# Mark's Example

(1) Fill in the chart to create a wellness baseline of where you are today versus where you would like to be in a year.

Date: February 2019

| Wellness Ethic | Current | Ideal | Gap |
|---|---|---|---|
| Love | 7 | 10 | -3 |
| Mind | 6 | 10 | (-4) |
| Body | 7 | 10 | (-3) |
| Spirit | 6 | 10 | (-4) |
| Relationships | 8 | 10 | -2 |
| Personal Pursuits | 7 | 8 | -1 |
| Professional Pursuits | 7 | 9 | -2 |
| Lifestyle Maintenance | 7 | 7 | 0 |
| **Observations** | | | |

*This is not a surprise. I'm writing this book because I need to be happier (mind) and more fulfilled (spirit). I also have an opportunity to lower my cholesterol levels to a healthy range (body).*

*I have a solid foundation to launch from—a loving family life and a great morning exercise routine. I'm looking forward to getting into this!*

# Choose Your Response
## to Life

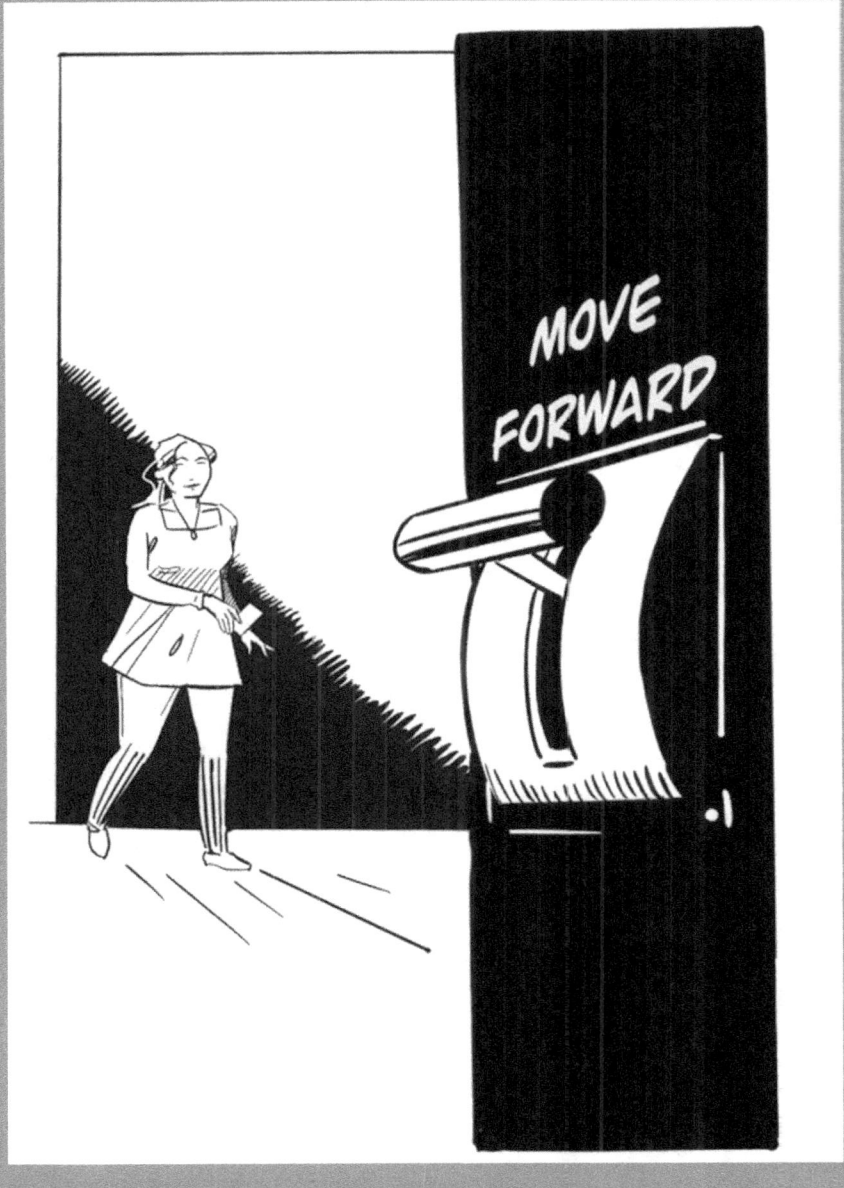

# CHAPTER 3

# A Story of Opportunity

It was a quiet Saturday night in downtown Charlotte. Most people were relaxing at home or out with friends, enjoying their time away from work. But I had different plans.

I parked my car on the street near the Bank of America corporate high-rise where my ninth-floor office was nestled. I felt the gravity of the moment as I stepped onto the sidewalk and took a deep breath of the refreshing forty-degree air, a most welcome gift from nature in the waning hours of January 2009.

I walked into the building and made obligatory eye contact with the guards. I felt self-conscious as I approached the security gate. I pressed my badge against the card reader, and the gate opened.

When I reached the elevators, I was relieved. I don't know if it's just me or if other people share my anxiety, but whenever I go through a security checkpoint, I feel uneasy, like I'm taking a test. If I earn the guard's trust, I pass the test and can proceed.

But getting up to my office was the easy part. The real test would occur when I completed my objective and left the building. How would I feel after the finality of my actions settled in? Would I lose my resolve, or was my trust in myself and the universe authentic?

The Great Recession bullied its way into my life in the fall of 2008. Before that time, I knew the housing market was imploding (I did work at Bank of America, after all). But my family and I lived comfortably in our house and had no intention of selling anytime in the next decade—I could ride out the down market. As for the volatility on Wall Street, my investments were earmarked for retirement, so I could patiently wait for the market to rebound.

And my job? The financial sector was a flaming mess, and no one was sure when it would bottom out. Despite that, Bank of America had a healthy balance sheet and was using that leverage to take advantage of the struggles of its competitors, like when it acquired Countrywide Financial and Merrill Lynch. All evidence suggested that Bank of America was well positioned to weather the recession without significant layoffs.

But even if they weren't, my layoff immune system was hearty: My work ethic was off the charts. I was a positive leader who did things the right way. And I was consistently rated "exceeds" in my performance reviews. If layoffs occurred, they would undoubtedly impact the other guy.

Throughout the fall, the recession continued to crater the US economy. Bank of America's stock steadily declined, and the Merrill Lynch acquisition unraveled as Bank of America's leaders lifted the hood on Merrill's financials and weren't enamored with what they saw.

As expected, the rumor mill kicked into high gear: Downsizing was on the table. It wasn't long before the stupidity began—a steady flow of layoffs occurred at levels above me, terminations that included deeply respected leaders. I felt exposed for the first time in my career and was worried that my job performance might not save me. It was unsettling. Though I wasn't passionate about my job—financial services wasn't my calling—I was passionate about providing for my family.

I talked with my wife about my fears. I knew the risk of losing my job was real since I was in a support function that wasn't essential to the bank's operations. The job market was dismal, so I could be unemployed indefinitely if I got the ax. I was also concerned about our finances—I didn't have a reserve built up that could withstand a loss of income for more than a few months without tapping into my retirement plan.

To make matters more alarming, our home was dropping in value as the housing market plummeted, and we were at risk of becoming upside down on our mortgage. Would we lose money if we had to sell our house because I lost my job and could no longer afford the monthly mortgage payments?

We decided to hedge our bets and put our house on the market. I also updated my resume and began to explore the job market aggressively. Work colleagues thought I was overreacting by taking these steps, but I didn't want to be in denial. I needed to respond to my circumstances in a way that would manage my risk. I had too much riding on it, namely, my family's well-being.

The storm clouds of professional doom drifted closer and closer to my livelihood with each passing day. Soon, the dark gray clouds hovered over my head—my job level was under evaluation!

My worst fears were confirmed when a friend with inside knowledge broke ranks and told me I was on *the list*. I then received a vague invitation for a Tuesday meeting with a senior leader. I knew that would be the day the dreaded Job Reaper would come a-knockin' at my door with a newly minted severance package in hand.

As I stood near my ninth-floor Bank of America office on Saturday night— just three more sunrises before D-Day (Downsizing Day)—I surveyed the dark, empty office floor. I was struck by the realization that it was a fitting metaphor for my lifeless financial services career.

I entered my office and began packing my belongings, filling boxes with files, binders, and personal effects. I occasionally paused to read old performance reviews and customer recognition letters from previous jobs. When I flipped through the Audrey and Emma file, which contained all the drawings and photos my children had me bring to the office over the years (so I would think about them at work), my heart was warmed. Bank of America no longer wanted my services, but my girls had always wanted me to be their dad. I couldn't think of anything more important than that, certainly not a job.

I felt a beautiful sense of peace when I finished packing. The universe had led me to this crossroads, and I surrendered to that. Losing my job during the Great Recession, when the housing market had imploded, job prospects were dim, and my family's financial safety net was frayed, should have stressed the hell out of me, or at least produced a facial tic or fifty. But it didn't.

After discovering my life was about to be upended, I doubled down on nurturing a positive mindset. I accepted my fate and framed my job loss as a gift that would compel me to take my life in a more fulfilling direction.

I recognize that viewing a layoff as a gift may seem odd, but I had a choice to make. Something stupid was about to happen—I was being let go. I could let a "woe is me" attitude settle in, blame others, and mope around. It would be an understandable reaction. But it would also undermine my ability to help my family recover from the disruption.

A more productive approach was to reframe my reality and make it perfect: The imperfect layoff was the perfect jolt that needed to happen at that precise moment in my life for me to break out of my career malaise. Framing it like that gave me hope and purpose, and proactively responding to my circumstances with positive energy was vital to successfully navigating the bleak housing and job markets.

With that healthy mindset in tow, I exited the elevator on the first floor of the Bank of America building with boxes in my arms. I now had to get past the guards. What would they be thinking? *That dude looks suspicious. He probably has gold bars in those boxes, stolen from the bank's vaults. Let's tackle him!*

Thankfully, my worrying was much ado about nothing, like it usually is. The guards were indifferent—I strolled to the exit without being flattened.

After I loaded the boxes into my car, I looked up toward my empty ninth-floor office—I was now professionally homeless. *This was really happening.* In three days, I would be unemployed and facing a very uncertain future.

But that was perfectly okay. I knew that *this too shall pass.* I trusted myself and the universe to figure out how to rebuild my life. My resolve was intact. I had passed the test.

On Tuesday, February 3, 2009, I was let go from Bank of America. After two months of unemployment, I had a job offer and a few more prospects trending favorably. I ended up accepting a position in Florida that better aligned with my career interests. I even sold my Charlotte house at a profit soon after starting the new job. Despite the economy being in the throes of a deep recession, I had defied the odds on practically every front.

I have no doubt that the results would have been very different had I not accepted the reality of my situation, reframed it as a perfect opportunity to reinvent myself, and chosen a proactive and empowering response that moved me forward.

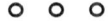

# CHAPTER 4

# Respond Perfectly to the Imperfect

## Imperfection Is Unavoidable, and That's Okay

As you live your life, expect imperfection. In fact, if you don't experience your fair share of false starts, stumbles, setbacks, goofs, embarrassments, curveballs, temptations, annoyances, do-overs, or even the occasional epic disaster, then you've accomplished something no one else has ever achieved. It's also thrilling news. It means you're immortal! If that's the case, invite your divine buddies over, tap the nectar keg, and let the festivities begin!

For the rest of us non-deities, imperfection is a familiar companion. How imperfection impacts you is more often the result of how you respond to it than the imperfection itself (ask a politician). When life challenges you, do you summon the wisdom and optimism of your Self-Actualized Genius and *intentionally respond* to your circumstances, based on what you control, to take your life in a positive direction? Or do you *impulsively react* in an emotionally charged way that undermines your interests and digs the hole deeper?

Imperfection will disrupt your blissful existence. It can come in the form of health, relationship, and job issues, daily struggles to eat well and exercise, and countless other challenges. Fortunately, there's a simple yet powerful approach that can help you choose your SAGe-inspired response to any obstacle (or opportunity) that crosses your path. Here's what it looks like in model form:

# Your
## Self-Actualized Genius

Accept → Frame → Respond = Best Outcome

The unifying force that holds the *Accept-Frame-Respond* model together is positive energy. Positive energy is the oxygen your SAGe breathes to maintain its mojo. You create positive energy when you acknowledge life as it is (*accept*) and develop a healthy perspective toward your circumstances (*frame*). You produce even more positive energy when you take love-centered action to move your life forward (*respond*). Positive energy and well-being go hand in hand. If you doubt that, try to think of a negative person who is thriving in their life. I've encountered many people who exude negative energy as their calling card. They never seem happy.

Negative energy chloroforms your SAGe. An incapacitated SAGe creates an opening for impulse to run amok in your life. When your impulse-

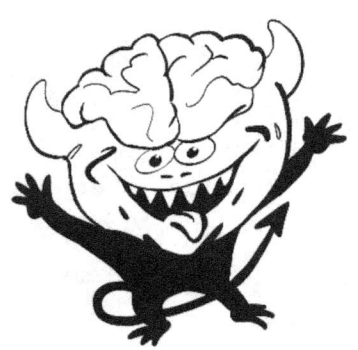

seized, self-sabotaging brain—which I'll call your "Mischief Mind"—is in charge, you ignore consequences in pursuit of pleasure and instant gratification. Your well-reasoned approach to life is muted when you enter mischief mode and follow through on your selfish and uninhibited urges with an attitude of *if it feels good, just do it (and damn the consequences!)*. Acting impulsively without considering the fallout often leads to poor decisions. We all have examples of when we impulsively said or did something we later regretted.

When you follow the Accept-Frame-Respond model, negative energy is neutralized, your Mischief Mind is sidelined, and your SAGe calls the shots. That doesn't always mean everything immediately gets better—especially after experiencing hardships like a job loss or the passing of a loved one—but it does mean you navigate through challenges by developing a healthy mindset and responding in ways that promote your well-being.

Let's take this empowering model for a spin.

## The Art of Accepting

Try to wrap your head around this paradox: Your life is imperfect, and that makes it perfect. Paradoxes can be mind-boggling sometimes. To unravel the meaning of this one, we'll start with a topic that has been debated throughout the ages, and when it's brought up as a conversation starter during a first date, it will reliably eliminate the possibility of a second date. As I'm sure you guessed, I'm referring to the nature of human existence.

A truth about human existence is that all humans who have ever taken an earthly breath—billions and billions of sentient beings—have lived their lives filled with dichotomous experiences: joy and suffering, struggle and ease, birth and death, and everything in between. There are no exceptions.

Understanding the nature of human existence, in all its unpredictable glory, is fundamental to acceptance. When you expect life to deliver both the desirable and undesirable, you are better positioned to surrender to the moment and accept your circumstances without judgment. If something unfortunate occurs, it isn't personal. You weren't singled out. The rational, accepting mind knows it can't wish away the stupid stuff and only embrace the good. Both are perfect representations of the way the world works.

**When you accept your circumstances with a productive mindset—coming to grips with the uncontrollable and finding peace within its limitations—you can begin to move forward.**

Consider the alternative of not accepting reality when something bad happens. Without healthy acceptance, your impulsive Mischief Mind can conjure up negative emotions like bitterness and anger, leading you to lash out at life. Or you can slip into the passive world of denial and avoid addressing what needs to be addressed. Just look at people in denial about substance abuse or domestic violence. Those situations desperately need to be authentically framed and urgently responded to. But without accepting that there's a serious issue, a person won't seek the help they need.

When you face difficulty, your SAGe is eager to tame your emotions and lead you to acceptance. An effective way to calm your mind and summon your SAGe is to utilize the *SAGe Deep Breathing Technique*. Here's the approach:

○ Find a comfortable and quiet place, private if necessary.

○ Close your eyes, place a hand on your belly, and slowly inhale through your nose—and deeply into your diaphragm—while silently repeating the words, "I am activating my SAGe." Feel your hand rise as your lungs fill to their maximum capacity.

○ Slowly exhale and feel serenity spread throughout your body.

○ Repeat the process until stress is reduced and negative emotions have abated. That will usually be the case after five to ten deep breaths. But take as long as required—getting to a peaceful state is worth it.

It may seem like deep breathing is too simple to make a difference, but its efficacy is supported by scientific research and how the autonomic nervous system (ANS) functions. In stressful times, your sympathetic nervous system—the branch of the ANS that prepares your body to react rapidly to threats (fight or flight)—becomes dominant. As a result, your heart rate, stress hormone levels, breathing rate, and anxiety levels rise, which can impair your logical reasoning ability.

Deep breathing activates your parasympathetic nervous system—the branch of the ANS that promotes relaxation—and suppresses your sympathetic nervous system. Once you're in a calmer, less reactive mindset, your clear-thinking SAGe can help you sort through the reality of what transpired and guide you to acceptance. Choosing acceptance doesn't necessarily mean you like what happened; it means you acknowledge what happened. You're positioning yourself to move forward.

If acceptance remains elusive, consider talking with a friend, a life coach, or a therapist. They can help you get there by offering an objective perspective or listening without judgment as you process your thoughts and emotions.

Another technique is to divert your mind. Go for a walk and connect with nature, watch a movie, clean your home, read, or listen to music. As your conscious mind focuses elsewhere, your emotions become less charged, and your subconscious mind works toward acceptance. When you distance yourself from a difficult situation, you often return to it with less stress, greater insight, and more optimism, which can lead to an acceptance breakthrough.

To sum up *acceptance*, I'll share an excerpt from "The Serenity Prayer" by theologian Reinhold Niebuhr. I love the profound wisdom of his words:

> *Grant me the serenity to accept the things I cannot change,*
> *the courage to change the things I can,*
> *and the wisdom to know the difference.*

## The Art of Framing

In post–World War II Japan, a group of railway engineers were challenged by their leaders to create a train that could travel twice as fast as existing trains. As a result of being given an audacious goal, the inspired engineers thought out of the box, stretched capabilities beyond perceived limits, and created the high-speed bullet train. The bullet train shattered locomotive speed records.

In the 1990s, GE's CEO, Jack Welch, latched onto "bullet train thinking"—setting audacious goals and challenging people to redefine what's possible—and mandated that every GE business think out of the box to drive down costs. I worked there at the time and was asked to join my department's "bullet train" team. Our bullet train challenge was to reduce our annual expenses by at least 10% without impacting headcount.

We scrutinized our expense budget and found enough opportunities to achieve our goal. I was a junior team member and made a respectable contribution. At the end of the project, we had a recognition luncheon where I was given a $50 gift certificate and a tin train Christmas tree ornament that looked like it was bought on clearance. The reward was appropriate for my contribution—as I *maturely* look back now—but, at the time, I was pissed. Oh boy, was I pissed! I expected more financial recognition based on my inflated view of my accomplishments.

After the luncheon, while sitting at my desk, my Mischief Mind framed the reward as a disrespectful act needing prompt correction. I thought: *Duh, of course I need to stomp to the executive sponsor's office and let him know what I think about his pathetic recognition!* I was confident that harsh feedback was the perfect response to deliver more recognition dollars.

So I marched to the executive's office with righteous indignation. I got more worked up with each irritated stride. *It's time to right this abomination!* I was primed for battle when I reached his office. Sparks were gonna fly!

He wasn't there.

Okay, I guess that was kind of anticlimactic. Deflated, I schlepped back to my desk. I calmed down and moved on with my day—I never got around to confronting the guy. Had I followed through on my outrage, driven by my absurd framing of the recognition, I would have received more money, but it would have been in the form of an unemployment check!

The *art of framing* starts with understanding that your experiences have no inherent meaning. They are neither good nor bad. Experiences are blank canvases devoid of sense until you add form, texture, and color to make them consequential. This empowers you to frame whatever happens to you in a productive light. You choose your reality by how you perceive your situation. Effective framing slams the door on negative perceptions in favor of a productive perspective that serves you. Like a vampire, negativity can appear at your door, but its destructive power is only unleashed if you invite it in.

There is a two-step process—*get underneath the truth* and *create a productive frame*—that you can use to frame what happens in your life to help you choose the best response.

## Step 1: Get Underneath the Truth

The first step—get underneath the truth—challenges you to sort through the noise to expose the essence of what has happened, not necessarily what you wish had happened. Ask yourself these questions to see if the truth emerges:

- What objectively happened, and why did it occur (root cause)?

- What was my contribution to the situation?

- What was in my control? What was out of my control?

- What did others contribute to what occurred?

- How would the most loving, nonjudgmental version of myself—my SAGe—want me to feel about what happened?

By understanding the truth, your framing and responding efforts become grounded in reality. You avoid setting unrealistic expectations or chasing after red herrings. You align yourself to serve the true needs that emerged from what transpired, whether it's the need to repair a relationship, address a health issue, give someone constructive feedback, or even focus on your own growth.

A common trap for people faced with a difficult situation is to blame others for their predicament. You may have to challenge yourself to avoid this tendency. Others may have had a role—perhaps even a dominant one—but usually there are other contributing factors, including the part you played.

As an example of getting underneath the truth, I'll offer an honest assessment from my life. Looking back at my Bank of America layoff years ago, I know the recession was a driving force. That was an external factor beyond my control. But when I shine the spotlight on myself, I realize I made myself vulnerable to a layoff by not nurturing relationships with influential leaders in my division. The truth is that I did bear some responsibility for my layoff, perhaps even the lion's share.

But sometimes the truth can be hard to capture, much like a stealthy cockroach that darts into a crevice once the kitchen light is turned on. In those cases, you must shine a brighter light and search every nook and cranny. The *5 Whys* approach can help. It was developed at Toyota and used by their employees to move past the symptoms of business problems to get to the root causes. When you employ the 5 Whys, you ask "why" multiple times until you get to the heart of what drove an issue. It usually takes about five iterations.

To illustrate, here's a challenge I need to work on: Sometimes I think the sky is falling and get upset when something minor goes wrong, such as an appliance breaking down or a computer program acting up.

○ *Why?* I feel overwhelmed and stressed in the moment.

○ *Why?* I lose perspective on what matters in life and what is trivial.

○ *Why?* I get angry rather than calmly framing and responding to frustrating situations.

○ *Why?* I haven't been meditating to bring peace into my life.

○ *Why?* I haven't made practicing spirituality a habit. (root cause)

Once you understand the truth of what happened, you can infuse that reality-based perspective into creating a productive frame.

## Step 2: Create a Productive Frame

When you create a productive frame, you nurture a positive mindset that interprets what has happened through a life-affirming lens. You bring out the best within you—your values, optimism, and love—and allow those virtues to shape how you perceive your circumstances so you can move forward with positive energy. Here are examples of positive and negative frames:

### REJECTED AFTER INTERVIEWING FOR A JOB

○ Positive Frame: *Although I didn't get the job, I got to practice interviewing. I learned about my strengths and development needs, and I'll apply what I learned moving forward. Sometimes it's a numbers game. I am talented. I will find the right job!*

○ Negative Frame: *I'm not talented enough when I compare myself to other applicants. There are hundreds of people applying for each job. It's impossible. I'll never get the job I want.*

### END OF A ROMANTIC RELATIONSHIP

○ Positive Frame: *Not all relationships work out. I know that my transition may be challenging—that's expected—but I'm committed to learning from the experience and focusing on self-care. I will find a loving partner who values my authentic self. I deserve to be loved!*

○ Negative Frame: *I will never find the right partner because there aren't good people out there. Maybe something is wrong with me?*

You'll notice with the positive frames that they don't include excuses or blame others. They're optimistic and realistic. They focus on learning from experiences and leveraging a person's strengths to move forward. The negative frames are defeatist. They are based on limiting beliefs and encourage inaction—why bother moving forward when you know it won't turn out well?

Limiting beliefs impact most people to some degree, including me. Limiting beliefs are a person's self-sabotaging thoughts about themselves or how life works. These deeply ingrained beliefs create a mental hindrance to success and are often influenced by past experiences and how someone perceives the world around them. Limiting beliefs are usually rooted in fear or irrationality—*I'm not smart enough, I'm too old, I'll never change, I always screw up, I don't deserve happiness, I'll never be successful.*

Uncovering limiting beliefs can be difficult. It requires you to get to the root cause of what's driving your beliefs and behaviors (5 Whys can help). But if you notice that you're treading water in life or find yourself repeating the same mistake over and over again, a limiting belief may be the culprit. Has a dream drowned in a flood of flimsy excuses because you don't believe you're talented enough to succeed? Do you resist adopting healthy habits, like eliminating junk food from your diet, because you falsely believe you don't have the willpower to overcome temptation? Do you fear relationship commitment because you think the other person will eventually reject you?

One of the best ways to eradicate a limiting belief is to expose its fallacy through logic. Is the limiting belief really true? Are there examples where it isn't? Then, consider alternative ways of thinking—how would your life-affirming SAGe reframe your belief so it reflects you at your best? Think along those lines and get excited about what could be possible. The light will begin to shine through. You'll be on your way to shifting your mindset.

| Limiting Belief | Reframed, Positive Belief |
|---|---|
| I don't have enough time to pursue my dreams. | There is plenty of time to move forward with my dreams if I say "no" to lesser priorities so I can say "yes" to what truly matters to me. I will prioritize pursuing my dreams, even if I take baby steps at first. |
| I can't advance in my career because I'm unwilling to devote my entire life to work. | Countless people have rewarding careers and maintain life balance. I will talk to people I respect to see how they juggle the demands of their careers and personal lives. Life balance is well within my capabilities. I will solve this! |
| I never stick to my resolutions. I just don't have the willpower. | Of course I'm capable of sticking to my resolutions. Billions of people have adopted changes in their lives. I'll try the techniques I learn in "The Wellness Ethic" and will be persistent as I move forward. I will be successful! |

If you struggle to construct a productive frame when faced with a challenge, imagine how you would want a friend to frame things in a positive light if they were in the same boat as you. Then, adopt that frame. Detaching yourself from the situation—as if you're an impartial observer—helps you push aside negative emotions and limiting beliefs that cloud your mental clarity.

It can take effort to hone your framing skills—it requires you to challenge preconceived notions as you put what happens in your life through a productive lens. But it'll soon become second nature. When you frame, remember to be realistic and truthful, but don't be shy about being bold in your framing assertion. After all, it is your reality. You choose it. You own it.

**Once you embrace being the master of your reality, you won't be willing to yield that empowering birthright to anyone or anything.**

*Finish each day and be done with it. You have done what you could. Some blunders and absurdities no doubt crept in; forget them as*

*soon as you can. Tomorrow is a new day. You shall begin it serenely*
*and with too high a spirit to be encumbered with your old nonsense.*
　—Ralph Waldo Emerson, American philosopher

# The Art of Responding

I was first exposed to the power of intentionally choosing your response to life when I read Viktor Frankl's seminal masterpiece *Man's Search for Meaning.*

Frankl, born in 1905, was a practicing psychiatrist in Austria as Nazi Germany began its evil aggressions during World War II. In 1942, he was arrested by the Nazis and then held as a prisoner in a series of concentration camps.

What he was subjected to during that time is unthinkable to all of us who didn't experience the Holocaust firsthand. But for a moment, try to imagine what it would be like to suffer from starvation to the point that your body begins to devour itself. You endure constant beatings. You work nonstop in the freezing winter with tattered clothes and shoes. You live with the constant fear that you could be sent to the gas chambers. On top of that daily horror, you have no idea whether your loved ones are still alive and, if they are, what torturous conditions they must endure.

Now imagine living like that for years with no sense of what the next hour will bring. That was Frankl's life from 1942 until he was liberated from Nazi imprisonment in 1945. That was the life of millions during the Holocaust.

Despite the horrific conditions, Frankl found that it was still possible to nurture a spiritual life. He and others could "retreat from their terrible surroundings to a life of inner riches and spiritual freedom." As Frankl wrote in *Man's Search for Meaning*:

*Everything can be taken from a man but one thing: the last of*
*the human freedoms—to choose one's attitude in any given set of*

*circumstances, to choose one's own way. And there were always choices to make. Every day, every hour, offered the opportunity to make a decision, a decision which determined whether you would or would not submit to those powers which threatened to rob you of your very self, your inner freedom; which determined whether or not you would become the plaything of circumstance.*[1]

That passage best captures your challenge when faced with a difficult situation: How can you respond to your reality in a way that stays true to the meaning of your life, to feel and share love? How can you avoid becoming the "plaything of circumstance"?

Whether you face significant challenges, or minor issues that pitter-patter into your life each day, **you are always empowered to choose a life-affirming response to your circumstances to move your life forward.**

You're not guaranteeing an outcome when you choose your response—the result is out of your control. You're putting yourself in a position for the best possible outcome given your situation—that's what you can control.

A paradigm shift regarding how you view outcomes may be required for you to become fully satisfied with your life. Most people view outcomes as pass/fail: I will take *X action* to accomplish *Y goal.* If they fall short of their goal, they feel like they've been unsuccessful.

When responding to life, the only outcome you should seek is to have your Self-Actualized Genius engage in the moment to move your life forward in a positive direction to the best of your ability. Nothing more, nothing less. If the result turns out favorably, that is preferred but not required for success, as the outcome can depend on factors outside your sphere of influence. A fulfilled life is an engaged life that brings out your best, based on what you can control, not necessarily a life filled with accomplishments that awe society.

US President Theodore Roosevelt captured the notion of an "engaged life" when he delivered "The Man in the Arena" speech at the Sorbonne in 1910:

> *It is not the critic who counts; not the man who points out how the strong man stumbles, or where the doer of deeds could have done them better. The credit belongs to the man who is actually in the arena, whose face is marred by dust and sweat and blood; who strives valiantly; who errs, who comes short again and again, because there is no effort without error and shortcoming; but who does actually strive to do the deeds; who knows the great enthusiasms, the great devotions; who spends himself in a worthy cause; who at the best knows in the end the triumph of high achievement, and who at the worst, if he fails, at least fails while daring greatly, so that his place shall never be with those cold and timid souls who neither know victory nor defeat.*

There are several factors to consider when choosing a response to what happens in your life, including:

○ Does my response align with my *values*?

○ Does my response have the potential to *move me forward* in a positive, loving direction based on what I control?

○ Am I comfortable with the *risk* of my response not working?

○ When possible, does my response have the potential to create a *win-win* for everyone involved? (A SAGe aspires to generate love throughout the universe.)

Ultimately, you're looking to thread the needle by choosing a response that answers "yes" to all four questions. Here's a visual of a decision-making process that captures those key questions. But full disclosure: This model has been certified as a doozy!

## Wellness Ethic Decision-Making

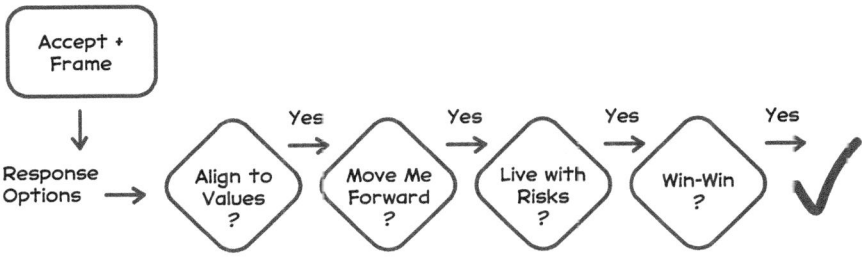

The Wellness Ethic Decision-Making model starts with accepting what has happened in your life and creating a positive frame. At this point, you have nurtured a productive perspective and are ready to choose your response. After identifying a potential response, test it against the four key questions. If a question weeds out a response, start the process again and continue testing responses until you find one that you can commit to.

Choosing a positive, loving response to life requires intentionality. The more you intentionally draw out the best within you, your Self-Actualized Genius, the more satisfying your life will be. That's because you already possess the awareness, know-how, and will to manifest a good life (even when stupid things happen)—you just have to activate those superpowers and take action.

Deciding to promote wellness in your life is a binary choice. You can exercise when your Mischief Mind wants to browse social media, eat a healthy meal when fast food is more convenient, and repair a relationship when your pride wants to dig in its heels. But sometimes our stubborn brain resists. If you struggle to make the right wellness choices, the next section in this book—"Adopt Change in Your Life"—will give you plenty of approaches to help you leap over the hump.

# Accept-Frame-Respond Model in Action

To illustrate how the Accept-Frame-Respond model is used in real situations, I'll share two examples from my life. The first one demonstrates my SAGe using the model correctly. The second represents my Mischief Mind calling the shots, which resulted in a total collapse of my mental faculties.

## MY CAREER (SAGe-DRIVEN RESPONSE)

Some of my friends and colleagues have advanced further in their careers than me. That can make me feel inadequate.

| Accept | Frame | Respond |
|---|---|---|
| Some people will advance further in their careers than me; some will not. That's a part of normal variation. | I'm not competing with anyone. I've lived a unique life on my terms based on what I could control. I've been successful enough to provide for my family. I've pursued my dreams. That's a full life by any reasonable standard. | My objective for the remaining five to ten years of my career is to continue to grow and add value. I will seek fulfillment with my corporate work, serve my life purpose, and pursue side hustles with passion. That's what I control. |

MY MENACING CAT (MISCHIEF MIND-DRIVEN RESPONSE)

My Savannah kitten, Queen Isabella of Castile, wakes me up by attacking my feet under the covers. I need my beauty sleep!

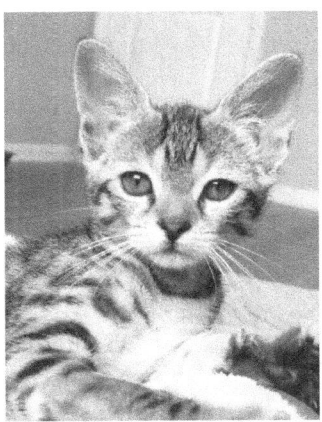

| Accept | Frame | Respond |
|--------|-------|---------|
| I accept that kittens will chase anything that moves. It's in their DNA. It's how they learn to hunt and survive. | I'm sorry, but there's no positive frame for this! My kitten is a demon beast sent from the lowest depths of the nether-world to disrupt my sleep! Argh! | I have no choice but to surrender to a two-pound kitten, and I will pray that she won't gnaw off one of my limbs! Oh, and I also think that I'll wake up my wife and ask her to amuse the ferocious feline so I can sleep. That seems like a good idea. |

o  o  o

## Move Forward on Your Wellness Ethic Journey!

(1) To apply the concepts from this chapter to your life, select a challenge you are dealing with and use the Accept-Frame-Respond model to choose a SAGe-inspired response to move your life forward.

| | Moving Forward |
|---|---|
| Describe your **challenge**. | |
| What does **acceptance** mean to you? | |
| How will you **frame** your challenge? | |
| What will be your SAGe-inspired **response?** | |

(2) Advanced Topics (going beyond the 80/20): Research "acceptance and commitment therapy" and "cognitive behavioral therapy" to explore advanced techniques that can help you take the Accept-Frame-Respond model to another level.

# Mark's Example

(1) To apply the concepts from this chapter to your life, select a challenge you are dealing with and use the Accept-Frame-Respond model to choose a SAGe-inspired response to move your life forward.

| | Moving Forward |
|---|---|
| Describe your **challenge**. | *I'm struggling to let go of my bitterness toward a former associate who screwed me out of $7,000 in a business venture. My negative self-talk is making me unhappy.* |
| What does **acceptance** mean to you? | *I accept that people do stupid things sometimes. I also accept that I won't be getting the money back.* |
| How will you **frame** your challenge? | *What he did was wrong, but it is out of my control. I pursued legal remedies to no avail. There's no point in passing judgment since I'm not walking in his shoes. It's best to accept what happened at face value, learn from it (I could have been more cautious), and move forward. Besides, the business venture was still very successful despite this setback.* |
| What will be your SAGe-inspired **response**? | *Simply move on with my life and put this episode in my wake. If I think about the issue, I will shift my focus to a positive thought. I refuse to let negative energy carry forward. I will also work on eliminating other negative self-talk in my life to boost my happiness.* |

# Adopt Change in Your Life

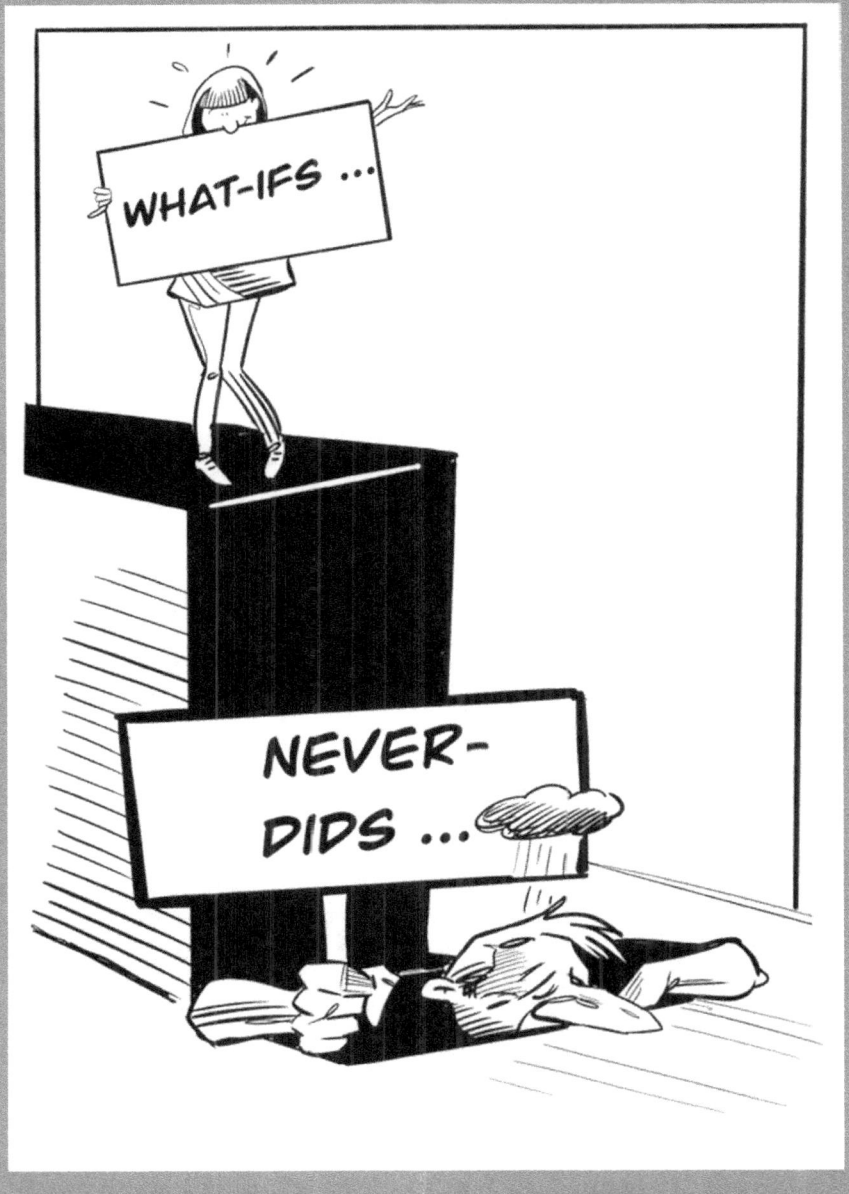

# CHAPTER 5

# A Story of Dreams

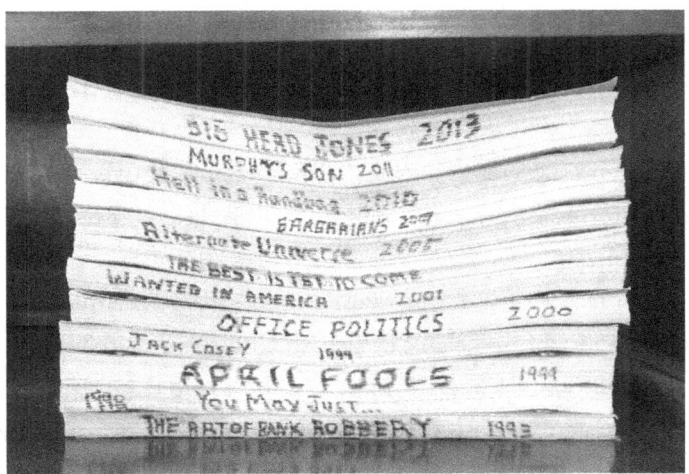

I desperately wanted to make it as a screenwriter. It became an obsession after I graduated from college. The comedies I wrote, captured in the picture above, represented a dream of Hollywood riches.

But it was the wrong dream.

Poorly executed.

For twenty years, I wrote screenplays as a side hustle. I thought every script I wrote would be the one that sold. Then reality would stomp on my dream and jolt me out of my "destiny is calling" reverie.

Once I finished a script and tried to market it, I became a crash test dummy as I collided head-first with a cement wall called the Hollywood gatekeeper. I tried every imaginable approach to get my writing into the hands of a decision-maker. I entered screenwriting contests that offered exposure. I sent query letters to agents, producers, studios, and talent. I tried to connect with people who knew people in the business, hoping they would be the conduit to get my work to an insider. But the gatekeeper was unmoved by my charms and persuasions.

On the rare occasion when my script did go out to an industry pro, I knew I had just bought a ticket to ride on an emotional Tilt-A-Whirl that would keep my head spinning for months until they rendered their verdict. Despite the staggering volume of ego-bruising rejection I received, I stayed in the arena.

There were high points along my screenwriting journey that gave me hope that I was on the verge of a breakthrough. My dream went into overdrive when I signed a contract with an agent. It overheated when a producer expressed interest in one of my screenplays—I was one call away from selling a script!

Or the time I won the top prize in a national screenplay contest—a full scholarship to a film school in British Columbia. What an insane life decision my wife and I had to make. At the same time as winning the scholarship, I received a promotion at GE. We also had a young daughter, were considering having another child, and had financial obligations to factor in, including a mortgage and car loans.

Should I have heaved caution to the wind, gone to film school, and trusted that my wife and I would find a way to make it work? Or was being risk-averse and staying at GE the better option? Putting it all on the line was the more celebrated path. There are thousands of movies with that very plot: The hero sacrifices everything to chase an audacious dream and then achieves glory through the sheer force of their will.

Sorry to disappoint. We declined the scholarship, which was one of the most painful decisions we ever made. We weren't willing to assume the financial risk of uprooting our lives so I could attend film school.

My wife regrets that decision to this day. I don't. My dreams are vitally important to me—they are my lifeblood in many ways—but I don't have tunnel vision when I dream. I also must provide for my family and help secure their future. That requires financial discipline and risk management. In a perfect world, my dreams would satisfy my financial needs, and that's a great life strategy. Unfortunately, it's not always feasible based on life circumstances. I thought the balanced decision was to continue with my corporate career while writing screenplays as a side hustle. I believe we made the right call.

I ended my screenwriting pursuits in my mid-40s when an odd opportunity to launch an internet start-up appeared out of the ether, but I'll get to that in a later chapter. When I stopped screenwriting, I felt like a failure. I didn't achieve my dream—I never sold or optioned a script. I couldn't even say I fully enjoyed the ride—it was filled with heartbreak.

Today, as I look at my screenwriting experience through the Wellness Ethic lens, I frame it much differently. Success wasn't really about selling a script—that was an outcome beyond my control. Success was about being in the arena, going on an adventure, and realizing my full potential as a screenwriter. It was about deriving joy from creative writing and having my artistic expression come alive with inspired energy. I didn't always dance with my muse, but it was a blissful tango when I did. I know now that it was a blessing to write screenplays.

But even when I reframe my dream with a positive spin, a part of me is still unsatisfied—I never wrote a script that fully reflected the passion and talent I had within me. That's my truth, and I have to own it.

At the time, I knew that breaking through in the film industry was a game of inches. If I didn't master the screenwriting craft, I wouldn't have a realistic shot. To take my writing to the next level, I needed to write more and learn more, which would require me to be all-in on my dream.

I was mostly-in.

Don't get me wrong—I was committed to writing screenplays. Completing a dozen in twenty years attests to that. I did most of my writing on weekends and vacations, with short periods of inactivity sprinkled throughout the years. But that level of commitment wasn't enough to reach my full potential.

Some suggest that to master a skill to the level of becoming elite, you must practice for at least ten thousand hours. Whether that's precisely true is up for debate, but I don't think the exact number of hours matters. The general concept is logical: The more you commit to a dream, the more likely you'll ascend to your fullest potential. Nonetheless, I still like the ten-thousand-hour benchmark—at least when applied to mastering advanced skills like screenwriting, playing the piano, or becoming a world-class athlete—so I'll use it.

With screenwriting, I estimate that I put in around seven thousand hours, which was well below the ten-thousand-hour threshold. Undoubtedly, the 30% gap adversely impacted my growth as a writer. Putting in ten thousand hours would have required adopting the habit of writing *every single day*, rain or shine, whether I was discouraged or inspired, exhausted or energized, focused or distracted.

I also fell short in learning the advanced techniques of the screenwriting craft. I did a lot to climb the learning curve, including taking classes, reading books, and joining writing groups. But did I dissect the top one hundred screenplays ever written to unlock their secrets? That would have been a game changer. Regrettably, I didn't do that. To plow through such a prodigious objective would have required adopting the habit of continuous learning *every single week*, rain or shine, whether I was discouraged or inspired, exhausted or energized, focused or distracted.

I knew at the time that I needed to change my habits to grow as a screenwriter. But I didn't develop a plan to do so. I didn't find the inspiration and motivation to boost my level of commitment. And I had a lot riding on it. Damn. My career path could have been radically different. *What if?*

I can't undo the past.

But I can learn from it.

I've applied the lessons from my screenwriting experience to *The Wellness Ethic* project. With my book, I define my dream by what I control: publishing a book representing my best attempt to articulate my vision, not how many books I sell.

I utilized practices in the next chapter (visual management, master habits, gamify change adoption) to help me adopt a two-hour writing habit in the morning before work. This supplements the bulk writing I do on weekends and vacations. Writing is what I do *every single day*, rain or shine, whether I'm discouraged or inspired, exhausted or energized, focused or distracted.

I also dedicate time each week to learning the craft of writing a non-fiction book by reading blogs and reference guides, analyzing successful books, and working with editors and beta readers.

When I finish *The Wellness Ethic*, I won't look back and wish that I could "undo the past." I will be fulfilled knowing that I nurtured the wonderful gift of my existence by being all-in on my dream.

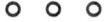

# CHAPTER 6

# Jack of No Change, Master of None

You are what you do, and about 45% of what you do is habitual, according to a Duke University study.[1] This means that almost half of your everyday actions are based on a preordained, habitual reaction to a trigger rather than a reasoned response that you apply to the moment. If you haven't designed your habits to nurture the wonderful gift of your existence, then a meaningful portion of your life may fall short of what you deserve.

How someone creates a habit is explained by the inner-workings of the brain. At the risk of oversimplification and, consequently, receiving reams of hate mail from the neuroscience community (which is not a community to trifle with, though it's not as bad as trifling with the beekeeping community), I'll describe how habits form in layperson's terms.

In Charles Duhigg's book *The Power of Habit*, habit formation is depicted as a habit loop with four elements:

o *Cue*: a trigger that occurs (feeling bored)

o *Craving*: the desire for a specific reward once the cue appears (wanting stimulation)

○ *Routine:* the action that responds to the cue and craving (playing a game on your phone)

○ *Reward*: the benefit of completing the routine (feeling engaged)[2]

When you repeat the cycle of experiencing a cue, consistently responding to the cue, and then receiving a reward, your brain forms neural pathways that link the cue with the routine. Soon, your brain will activate a craving when the cue appears, compelling you to follow the routine to get the reward. As the brain's neural pathways strengthen with each cycle repetition, you can find yourself automatically doing the routine whenever the cue occurs, almost without thinking—like grabbing your phone to check email after you wake up. Your routine will have become a habit.

Habits are the brain's way of conserving energy to free up cognitive resources for more complex activities. They also make life efficient—imagine what it would be like if you had to fully engage your conscious mind with every habitual activity you perform, such as driving a car or brushing your teeth. Habits can improve your life, provided they promote well-being. But sometimes your habits aren't healthy.

So, how do you break a bad habit? You guessed it. You respond in a healthy way to cues and cravings (instead of eating junk food to relieve stress, go for a walk), get a reward (feel relaxed), and then repeat that healthy cycle over and over again. This forms new neural pathways and creates a good habit.

The brain's ability to create and strengthen neural pathways is called neuroplasticity, and neuroplasticity is empowering. It enables your brain to learn new things and develop new thinking patterns. Your brain can adopt healthy behaviors and break the not-so-awesome ones. This translates to an enormous capacity for change.

Let's take it a step further. Your brain controls your choices and perception of your experiences—your brain shapes your life. Since your brain is not set in its ways, your life is not set in its ways. I don't think I emphasized that point adequately. I'll try again.

# YOUR LIFE IS NOT SET IN ITS WAYS!

Perhaps I should jack up the font size to emphasize this liberating fact. Heck, I'll even add more exclamation points in case the concept is not landing.

# YOUR LIFE IS NOT SET IN ITS WAYS!!!

You are capable of steering your life in a different direction. *Adopting change is in your wheelhouse.*

## Adopting Change Ain't Easy, but It Can Be Easier

Change comes in many forms. To keep it simple, we'll consider two types of change: habitual and structural. Habitual changes involve incorporating repeatable behavior into your everyday life (morning meditation, afternoon stretching). Structural changes represent a recalibration that pivots you in a new direction (begin a new job, start a family). Change, no matter what form it takes, can have a positive, negative, or neutral impact on your well-being.

Being adept at adopting positive change is a vital skill that helps you get the most out of your life. However, the changes you attempt to make—whether initiated by you or in response to external events—can be challenging to adopt, no matter how compelling the case for change is.

Consider the lifestyle modification study published in the *Journal of the American Medical Association* in 2013. This sobering research showed that patients who had coronary heart disease or suffered a stroke struggled to make essential lifestyle changes to improve the quality of their lives.[3] For the three most important changes—quitting smoking, adopting a healthy diet, and engaging in regular exercise—14.3% of the patients didn't change behaviors in any of the three areas, and only 4.3% improved in all of them.

Imagine your life being on the line, and you are faced with a binary choice: Change your lifestyle to improve the quality and longevity of your life, or continue with the status quo and further erode your health. It would seem to be an easy choice since the upside of changing your lifestyle should trump all other considerations. However, the data shows that people can struggle to translate reason and desire into lasting change, no matter what's at stake.

Take a moment to reflect upon your relationship with change:

○ What habits do you currently have, both good and bad?

○ Are there changes you'd love to make that would enhance your life? Do you feel confident you could make those changes? Why?

○ What have been your keys to success in adopting meaningful change? Does anything hold you back?

What did this exercise tell you about yourself? If you're like many people, you probably have a handful of good habits and have made lasting changes in your life. That's important because it gives you a foundation of practices and lessons learned to anchor your growth. But you probably also have a bad habit you'd like to curb and a pivot or two you'd like to make. You may even be baffled: You want to behave differently, so why don't you *just do it!*?

Unfortunately, you can't order a vial of magic pixie dust on Amazon and wish your life into a fairy-tale existence. It takes hard work. It requires adopting change. And we know change ain't easy. But it can be easier if you're intentional with how you approach it. We'll learn how.

# Never Let a Good Opportunity to Create a Model Go to Waste

You had to see this coming. By now, you should know that I like to build models to simplify things. It's how I roll. Someday, I may create a model to show people how to create models. But that would be obnoxious to humanity, so I probably shouldn't do that. Nonetheless, here's a model that can help you adopt change in your life:

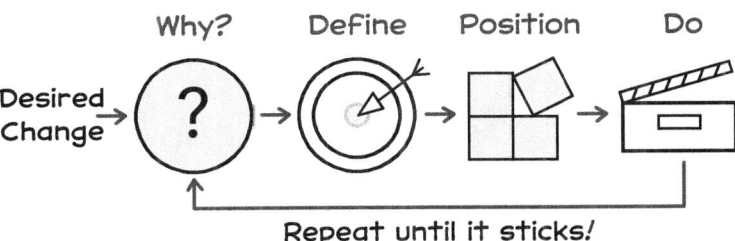

You significantly increase the odds of adopting change if you are inspired by your reason for seeking the change (*why*), identify your desired outcomes (*define*), set yourself up for success (*position*), and maintain an optimistic and resilient mindset as you incorporate the change into your life (*do*).

Before we go deeper into the model, think about a change you want to make. As you read the rest of this chapter, consider how the insights and approaches could help you adopt the change. Then, make it happen!

## **Why?** – Define – Position – Do

It's always a good idea to understand *why* you're doing something before you do it, whether it's getting married, changing jobs, or, as I did decades ago, making a split-second decision on a highway to let a stray cinder block pass under your car (rather than driving around it). Spoiler alert: Driving over a cinder block causes it to get stuck in the car's undercarriage, which then disables the vehicle and creates a traffic jam as the idiot driver waits for a tow truck.

We've heard the saying "think before you act" since childhood, but do we reliably follow that wisdom? Are we intentional with our responses to life—using our reasoned mind to make decisions—or do we let emotions and irrationality get in the way? We'll explore a scenario that can challenge people—adopting an exercise habit—to understand the dynamics at play.

Some people begin a new exercise regimen with guns blazing, only to have their enthusiasm wane in a few days. It's a novel routine that requires effort to turn into a habit. And exercise is not always fun, especially when you begin.

Once the impulsive Mischief Mind senses vulnerability, it lunges toward its prey. In the moment of truth—when the person is deciding whether to exercise—their Mischief Mind could remind them how cozy their bed is, how tired they are, or how cold it is outside. The Mischief Mind doesn't give a damn about why you should exercise. It wants low-effort gratification now!

Does your SAGe stand a chance against the manipulative Mischief Mind? Absolutely. That is, provided your SAGe is armed with *an inspiring why that reflects how your life will improve if you promote well-being.* A why so meaningful that it's top of mind when you're in the heat of battle and deciding to commit or retreat. When your why is that compelling, your Mischief Mind cowers in submission, and intention crushes impulse.

You'll build an exercise habit if your SAGe regularly defeats your negative impulses when deciding to work out. When I started exercising, I reminded myself of my why: I needed to be healthy to thrive in my life, set an example for my children, and live long. My why inspired me to cement my exercise habit. Today, I don't think about why I exercise—I just do it.

Connect with the whys in your life and let them motivate and inspire you to do what your SAGe knows you should do. Your whys could center around yourself—being healthier and more energetic, feeling love, achieving an important objective, being happier, finding inner peace, feeling proud, living a dream. Or they could be external in nature—inspiring someone, supporting others, making the world a better place.

## Why? – **Define** – Position – Do

Once you know why you should do something, the next step is to define what success looks like—what are your desired outcomes? In business, a common practice is to establish SMART goals. That is, goals should be Specific (clearly defined), Measurable (quantifiable), Achievable (doable), Relevant (aligned with what's important to you), and Timely (time-bound). SMART business goals are designed to motivate employees to rally around clear objectives and help managers gauge how well their teams perform against defined criteria.

But what about utilizing SMART goals in your personal life? At times, they can be beneficial. If, for example, you have a serious medical issue and need to modify your lifestyle to get well, then you'll want to be very specific about the changes you need to make. SMART goals—that you take seriously—could save your life. Examples of SMART wellness goals are walking 10,000 steps a day and meditating for ten minutes at least five times a week.

But there is a downside to SMART goals—the rigid structure can stifle flexibility and cause undue stress. Here's how I approach setting objectives:

*I avoid the trap of overcommitting.* Setting too many objectives can be overwhelming and make you unhappy. You probably won't even be successful—when you try to do too much, you rarely do much at all.

*I view my objectives as intentions and not goals.* The word choice—intentions versus goals—fosters a subtle shift in my mind. It tells me to be flexible with what I set out to achieve. Life happens, and I need to adapt to the steady infusion of reality that will be introduced into my well-laid plans.

*I carefully consider the importance of my intentions before timeboxing them or creating a measurable outcome.* The more critical the intention, the more likely I'll be specific. For example, retiring from corporate America is a high priority to me, so I have set an intention to retire by sixty. My financial advisor and I have developed a year-by-year strategy to position me to do that, and we adjust as life happens. If I weren't specific with my plans, I wouldn't know what percentage of my income to save for retirement; I would be directionless on something important to my future well-being.

*When I set specificity to an intention, I ensure it is largely within my control.* Although I dream about how fun it would be if I were dealt a royal flush in my pursuits, I won't put my satisfaction in the dealer's hands. That's why, in my career, I haven't set specific targets around job titles or compensation—both are out of my direct control. I'll continue to position myself for growth as best I can and respond to the opportunities I attract. I can control that.

To provide examples of defining intentions, this is what I'm committed to as I write this chapter in 2022: publish *The Wellness Ethic* in 2025, lower my cholesterol to a healthy level by the end of 2022, and exercise an hour a day. These intentions feel right—they have strong whys and are within my control.

When you evaluate your intentions, you are doing something right if you're moving forward. Build upon that. If you're falling short, the rest of this chapter will give you a ridiculous number of approaches that can help you bring positive change to your life. Prepare to geek out on change adoption!

## Why? – Define – **Position** – Do

How well you position yourself for success often determines whether you adopt a difficult change. This step requires effort. But is the change worth it? There is no shortcut to greatness. However, greatness gets easier as you strengthen neural pathways and build your change adoption muscles.

Positioning for success involves developing an *execution plan* (rolling out the change) and a *strategy for adopting change* (ensuring the change sticks once it's rolled out). They work together. The effort you put in should be proportional to the challenge of adopting the change. If it's easy, then simply adopt the change. If not, then put in the time to position yourself for success and ratchet your effort based on what's required to be successful.

## Execution Plan

Imagine I issue a challenge. You have a bow and arrow in your hands, a burlap sack on the ground next to you, and a target forty-eight feet away. I will give you one shot to hit the bullseye from that distance. If you're successful, you win the burlap sack. Everyone can use a good burlap sack, and it's not every day that you get a chance to win one, so I'm confident this excites you.

Then imagine that the good news keeps coming: I will give you a month to take your shot, so you'll have ample time to hone your archery skills.

Forgive me, but I forgot to mention that the burlap sack contains ₹81 million Indian rupees (about $1 million). If you hit the bullseye, you'll also get to keep the loot, assuming that's your preference.

Given those circumstances, would you immediately shoot the arrow, hoping you somehow defy every conceivable odd on the planet and splinter the bullseye?

Or would you take the month I gave you and execute a plan to improve your archery skills? Would you take lessons and watch training videos? Would you practice, rain or shine, until your fingers bled? Would you dress up like William Tell, with an apple in your hand, and walk around town asking strangers if they would help you with your target practice? Of course you'd do stuff like that; well, maybe not that bizarre William Tell idea—not all of my ideas are winners—but the point is you would develop a plan to optimize your time over the next month to put yourself in the best position to succeed.

What if you put in all that hard work and still missed the bullseye? You would have no regrets because you would have hit the bullseye that *really* mattered: experiencing life with your SAGe at the helm, controlling what you can, and doing your best with what you cannot. Whether you hit the bullseye or not is almost immaterial to the bigger picture of your life journey. I say *almost* because—let's keep it real—winning a burlap sack would be really awesome no matter what journey you're on.

The effort you put into planning should align with your experience level and the challenge of your intention. The less experience you have, or the more challenging the objective, the more planning you should do.

Planning is the process of breaking down uncertainty and complexity into manageable steps so you know what you need and what path to follow to meet your objectives. As you plan, you build confidence. The lofty dream in the clouds descends to earth. You can touch it. Without planning, a person can be like a single-engine pilot flying without a navigation system on a foggy day.

Let's walk through an overly simplified example to illustrate the value of planning: You want to get your master's degree. That's a hairy undertaking. So, how do you break down that noble intention into manageable steps to make it accessible? You could build a basic plan with steps like: (1) research schools and degree programs, (2) determine schedules and time commitments, (3) sort through financing options, (4) complete the application process, (5) enroll in a school and finalize financial aid, and (6) take classes. Before you know it, you'll be on your way to earning your degree and supercharging your career!

**When you break down your intentions into manageable steps, the daunting transforms into the doable.**

*A journey of a thousand miles begins with a single step.*
—Lao-Tzu

The planning tools you use should vary based on what you're trying to accomplish. A simple to-do list may suffice for straightforward objectives. A list of tasks with milestones could be necessary if your undertaking is more involved. You may even need a full-blown project plan if you embark upon something ambitious, such as starting a business. Whatever approach you take, the moment you craft your plan, it ages—life happens; you learn more as you go. Evolve your plan accordingly to keep it relevant.

One common criticism of planning is that it slows progress. Some people almost regard their lack of planning as a badge of honor—they "get shit done" and react to what happens. I don't subscribe to that approach. I love to get things done. I also like to plan when it adds value. In my experience, I've found that planning and having a bias for action don't have to be at odds. Done correctly, planning points you in the right direction. It prevents false starts and rework. *You move more quickly and confidently when you plan effectively.*

If planning is not something you do for your significant intentions, ask yourself: Is it wise to shoot *before* you aim?

## Strategy for Adopting Change

Adopting meaningful changes in your life can be challenging. The more you proactively confront that reality, the more successful you'll be. I'll offer seven change adoption approaches that should provide plenty of practical options to help you get to the promised land of adopting change that stands the test of time. Attainment *without* sustainment is fleeting glory.

### 1. KEEP YOUR INTENTIONS IN FRONT OF YOU

When you are reminded about an intention, you receive a nudge to follow through on your commitment. By keeping the intention at the forefront of your mind, your SAGe will be activated to drive your actions.

**Visual management** is an effective approach to keeping your intentions front and center so you act in accordance with how you want to live your life. Visual management provides visual prompts that encourage people to align their thoughts and behaviors with a priority. In everyday life, it can be a "Maximum Capacity" sign in an elevator, messages on a bulletin board in a kitchen, or a "No Trespassing" sign on private property.

To illustrate how visual management could apply to your personal life, we'll go through an example: You want to hike for two weeks in majestic Alaska. You'll need to save money for the vacation, and your budget is tight. And don't forget about getting in shape because outrunning a Sasquatch in the rough Alaskan terrain requires you to be as svelte as a caribou. No, forget that last example. If you ran into a Sasquatch, the Sasquatch would just throw a big rock at your head, and you would be screwed no matter what shape you were in.

So, how could visual management help? You could create an inspiring screensaver showing Alaskan mountains so that whenever you log on to one of your devices, you're reminded of the financial sacrifices you need to make to take the trip. You could also create an eye-catching visual of a fundraising thermometer that shows your progress toward your trip savings target. Placing that on your refrigerator would remind you to watch what you spend.

Visual management doesn't have to be complicated. It could be a Post-it note stuck to your computer reminding you to do something. Have fun with visual management. Refresh it whenever it stops grabbing your attention.

## 2.   MASTER HABITS THAT MOVE YOU FORWARD

You have learned that 45% of what you do is habitual. Your SAGe wants that 45% to work for you. Becoming a master of your habits, rather than your habits mastering you, requires a mindful approach to habit building. Which habits can you create, expand upon, or eliminate to promote wellness? Which habits can you do in the morning, afternoon, or evening to further your intentions?

To excel at building habits, consider **stacking your habits.** One of the most effective ways to build a habit is to incorporate it into an established routine. Do you want to start practicing yoga? If you have already cemented the habit of exercising each morning, practice yoga after you exercise. Soon, yoga will become a natural extension of that morning routine.

Use **instigation habits** to make habit adoption easier. An instigation habit is a preparatory action or a cue that reduces barriers to completing a desired habit. For example, you could prep healthy meals on Sunday for the upcoming week (instigation habit—preparatory action) to make it easier to eat healthy (desired habit). Or place a book on your nightstand (instigation habit—cue) to remind you to read at night (desired habit).

**Practice habit substitution.** Substitute a good behavior for an unhealthy one. If you have a habit of drinking alcohol when stressed, meditate instead. Rather than spending hours on social media when bored, engage in a fulfilling hobby. Soon, you will form a good habit and crave its positive reward.

Another best practice is to **commit to regularly engaging in a good habit, even if it's brief due to other commitments**. That's how I approach exercising. My daily routine lasts about ninety minutes. Some days, usually because of work overload, I may exercise for ten minutes, but I'll keep the habit going.

And for those times when life takes over, **if you break your streak of engaging in a good habit, learn from the experience and try to avoid missing the next day**. If you feed a negative streak, it will crave another fix, and then another one after that. Before long, you will have developed a bad habit.

Be patient as you build your habits. It's acceptable to start small and build up over time. The key is to establish a reliable routine of action.

## 3. GAMIFY CHANGE ADOPTION

Modern games are addictive by design. Game designers deftly deploy reward systems, social influence tactics, early wins, constant feedback, dashboards, and dozens of other techniques to keep you coming back for more, even if that *more* can be, at times, a time-sucking drain on your productivity. Yet you still engage. Gamification is that powerful. You create a win-win scenario by turning that power toward something productive, like change adoption. You may even have fun as you increase your odds of adopting change. I'll share a few of my favorite gamification techniques:

**Set up a system of rewards and penalties.** An effective reward could be simple, like treating yourself to a night out if you finish your spring cleaning. Penalties could be something like the clichéd "put money in a jar" if you do something counter to your intention, such as getting worked up by current events (I would need a whiskey barrel to hold the coins). Whatever approach you choose, ensure it is motivating and that you'll hold yourself accountable.

**Utilize a checklist or a calendar to track progress.** Is there anything more gratifying on this planet than checking off an item on a to-do list? Checklists are effective in helping people stay focused on what they want to get done. Plus, you get the bonus of a little dose of dopamine (a brain neurotransmitter associated with pleasure) with each item you cross off your list. That's one way games keep you hooked—small achievements that make you feel good.

A calendar can also be an easy way to bring gamification into your life. Just print one off and mark an "X" on each day you honor your positive intention, such as walking two miles, refraining from junk food, or performing a random act of kindness. You'll soon have a streak that you'll want to keep alive. If you miss a day, start another streak and aim to beat your previous best.

**Leverage an app.** There are apps with nudging and gamification features designed to help you adopt new habits, break bad ones, and keep you focused on your intentions—there's an app for practically anything you want to achieve. And with advancements in artificial intelligence and behavioral sciences, apps are constantly improving. Search "gamify my life" on the internet, and you'll be flooded with options.

## 4. NURTURE A POSITIVE MINDSET

Positive thinkers have an optimistic attitude that good will come into their lives, and they spin a positive frame when it doesn't. Positive thinking plays a vital role in change adoption. You are more apt to move forward when you believe you can do something. You are more resilient when facing obstacles because you know you can overcome them.

> *The difference between a successful person and others is not a lack of strength, not a lack of knowledge, but rather a lack of will.*
> —Vince Lombardi, American football coach

When you have a negative mindset, you often don't get past "go." Why bother trying when you know you're going to fail? Or, if you muster enough courage to give it a shot, you're more likely to bow out at the first sign of trouble. After all, you knew it was too difficult, so you fulfilled your prophecy. Negativity is the foil of ambition. To boost positivity in your life:

**Use affirmations to create a steady drumbeat of positive reinforcement.** An affirmation is a positive statement about what you're committed to. When you repeat it regularly with conviction, you begin to believe what you're saying or have written. You *become* the affirmation in thought and action.

To craft an effective affirmation: (1) Make it personal (start the affirmation with the word "I"), (2) Use the present tense (as if it's already happening), (3) Be positive (focus on what you want to be or achieve, not what you want to avoid), (4) Be specific (clearly articulate what you're trying to manifest in your life), and (5) Be realistic (make it attainable so you foster belief).

In my case, each morning, I repeat ten spiritual affirmations that define who I am and how I want to go about my day. I have them as my computer background image, so I'm prompted to complete my affirmation habit when I turn on my computer. Here are a few of them: *I gratefully live in the now and am unbothered by the past or future. I let go of what I can't control and manage expectations accordingly. I surrender to the design of the universe; thus, I choose not to suffer. I understand there's a time for everything and all things pass. I commit to the Wellness Ethic, caring for mind, body, and spirit.*

**Visualize your success.** Many elite athletes utilize this technique to help achieve peak performance. To visualize your success, imagine succeeding at a task, and be very specific: What exactly are you doing, step by step? What are your surroundings? What do you hear? How do you feel? Then, replay that vivid sequence in your mind over and over again.

Visualizing your success boosts your confidence that you can achieve your objectives because you will have already experienced success in your mind dozens, if not hundreds, of times. Olympic slalom skiers, for instance, will visualize navigating the course they're about to ski—every gate and turn—until their success skiing down the slope becomes imprinted in their brains.

**Practice positive journaling.** The ancient Greek philosopher Socrates once said, "The unexamined life is not worth living." Socrates was known for being a rather intense fella. But the spirit of what he was saying is important.

Examining your life provides insight into what's working and what isn't. It can inspire your SAGe to shape how you accept, frame, and respond to your circumstances. *Positive journaling* can drive your examination process.

To develop the habit of positive journaling, establish a morning routine of listing your intentions for the day in a journal and visualizing your successful execution. At the end of the day, record in your journal your acknowledgment of the outcomes (accept), what you learned and your productive spin (frame), and your plan for moving forward (respond). Positive journaling strengthens your positive mindset and helps you tune your approach to life.

**Surround yourself with positive people, and move on from those who are not.** Positive people, through the example they set and the encouragement they readily give others, bring inspiring energy to everything they touch—their life force is contagious. Being around positive people motivates you to engage in life and be the best version of yourself.

Conversely, has a bad influence ever sent you down the wrong path, or has a naysayer broken your spirit? Negative people are negative because they're usually struggling in their own lives. Their negativity rarely reflects upon you and what you're trying to do. Remember that when someone attempts to drag you down—either ignore them, give them feedback and an opportunity to change, or move on and associate with positive people. If left unaddressed, negativity will claim squatter's rights on your consciousness.

## 5. ALIGN SUPPORT

You don't have to improve your life on your own. There is always someone out there who wants to help you. There is always someone trying to do what you want to do and would welcome camaraderie. Engage with those people. You'll increase your odds of success if you do. To align support:

○ **Tell your friends and family what you're working on and ask for their support.** Be specific about what you need from them. You may need ongoing encouragement and help with keeping temptation away. Or the support could be taking on a few of your responsibilities to create space for you to focus on your desired change.

○ **Engage with a mentor or a certified professional (doctor, therapist, dietitian, life coach, fitness trainer) who has experience with what you're trying to accomplish.** Partnering with someone with the expertise to help you chart a course and work through challenges can be invaluable. Seeking help is an admirable act of self-love.

○ **Find an accountability partner.** An accountability partner takes on the role of keeping you honest with your intentions. They celebrate your successes with you, help you when you struggle, and motivate you to move forward. For example, the arrangement could involve two friends trying to accomplish something and agreeing to support each other along the way, though the accountability relationship doesn't have to be reciprocal. Trust, commitment, and a willingness to be vulnerable are key aspects of a successful partnership.

○ **Join a group of like-minded folks.** Take a dance class. Participate in an online community. Join a gym or a club. Whatever approach you take, the more you surround yourself with people who do what you do, the more motivated you'll be to keep doing those things. Get immersed in the fun and dynamic world of your positive pursuits.

## 6. BE AUDACIOUS WITH YOUR ACCOUNTABILITY

This change adoption technique is my favorite. It can be a forcing function to encourage you to treat your intention as a top priority, not just in mind but in action. **What audacious reward or penalty can you create that will raise the stakes and give you almost no choice but to adopt the change you seek?**

Do you want ideas to get the juices flowing? How about this one: If you want to exercise regularly but can't seem to maintain a consistent routine, offer to take a friend out to dinner at the best restaurant in town whenever you miss your exercise intentions for the week. Or, if you want to eliminate a vice, promise a family member that you'll give them one of your paychecks if you fail.

## 7. ANTICIPATE YOUR DERAILERS AND ACT ON THAT INSIGHT

The boxer Mike Tyson famously said, "Everybody has a plan until they get punched in the face." If your change is meaningful, it probably won't be easy. There will be moments of truth when you'll have to decide to move forward or regrettably succumb to a loss of resolve. **Anticipate what could derail you and act on that insight.** How can you be proactive to put yourself in position for success? Setbacks are lurking—how can you neutralize them?

If you were giving up alcohol, what would you do when a friend wants to go to a bar? You could avoid the temptation and suggest doing something else together, like going to a movie. If coworkers order drinks at a company function and the waiter and everyone at the table look at you for your drink order, what do you say? By scripting your response in advance, you will be more likely to follow that script when you're put to the test.

Or, if you want to improve your diet but are tempted to "punch yourself in the face" by buying junk food when you go grocery shopping, what can you do proactively to increase the odds of making healthy choices? You could order online to limit impulse buying. You could research healthy snack options. Or you could avoid grocery shopping on an empty stomach.

I know that last example from experience. When I'm hungry and go grocery shopping, *everything* looks delicious, even circus peanuts. In case you've never had them before, circus peanuts are peanut-shaped marshmallow candies that originated in the nineteenth century. Through the dark magic of alchemy, they evolved into a weirdly textured, artificial-banana-flavored confection whose only usefulness to a civilized society is to serve as a biodegradable substitute for Styrofoam packing material. But on an empty stomach, yum!

## Position for Success Tool

To help you identify which change adoption techniques to use for a change you want to make, here's a tool that captures the seven best practices:

| Why | Define | Position | Do |
|-----|--------|----------|-----|

# Position for Success

- ☐ Keep your intentions in front of you.
- ☐ Master habits that move you forward.
- ☐ Gamify change adoption.
- ☐ Nurture a positive mindset.
- ☐ Align support.
- ☐ Be audacious with your accountability.
- ☐ Anticipate your derailers . . .

## Why? – Define – Position – **Do**

Now that you are intimate with why you want to change, have defined what success looks like, and have positioned yourself for success, it's time to make it happen. Just a minor technicality, right?

As you make significant changes in your life, you will experience challenges. Everyone does. But what successful people do that separates them from the pack is they DON'T GIVE UP!

They monitor their progress. They examine what's working and what's not, and adjust their approach accordingly. If they fall down, they stand up wiser from the experience. When they're successful, they celebrate.

As they move forward, they bring their SAGe to the party and choose their best response to the reality that comes their way. By doing so, they may need to alter their plans or try different tactics. They may need to go back to the drawing board and reexamine their why, redefine what success looks like, or try other change adoption approaches. It's a part of the process. But their stick-to-it-iveness will lead to better results. It will bring satisfaction to their lives.

Maintaining a positive mindset will be one of your keys to success as you adopt change. For the more difficult changes you undertake, transitioning from the "old you" to the "new you" can be an emotionally taxing process. But knowing that a transition is a process that's expected to have ups and downs is liberating. It tells you that the obstacles and setbacks you experience when making a significant change are perfectly normal. They don't represent failure. They represent a transition behaving like a transition. You can persevere.

The best depiction of the transition process I've come across is contained within William Bridges' classic book *Transitions: Making Sense of Life's Changes*. In the book, Bridges describes three natural stages of successful transitions: *endings, the neutral zone,* and *new beginnings.*[4]

The first stage—endings—is characterized by letting go of your old self. As you progress through this stage, you can feel frustrated at times or be in denial. You can also be sad and angry and experience other negative emotions as you come to grips with changing a part of yourself. After all, you're trying to let go of something familiar—it can be uncomfortable.

The next stage—the neutral zone—is an in-between stage where you go back and forth between your old self and the new you. You may be uncertain and impatient. Some days, you're living the desired change, which can energize you. On other days, you may revert to your old self and feel discouraged. But you'll soon find that the good days start to outnumber the not-so-good days, and you'll feel the tide turning as you build momentum.

The last stage—new beginnings—has you firmly planted in your new world. You've adopted the change and effectively transitioned to the new you.

Think about the meaningful transitions you have gone through, whether it was a breakup with a partner, moving to a new city, becoming a parent, or something else that impacted you. Did you go through the three transition stages? In retrospect, what worked well with your approach to the transition, and what would you have handled differently now that you understand the nature of transitions? Leverage those insights moving forward.

**You have it within you to be a successful change agent. It's how your brain was designed. Your capacity to change is a scientific fact!**

o o o

## Move Forward on Your Wellness Ethic Journey!

(1) List one change you want to make—big or small—and detail your change adoption strategy. Then, make it happen!

| | |
|---|---|
| **The Change:** Describe the change you would like to make. | |
| **Why?:** Why would you like to make the change? | |
| **Define:** Define what success looks like. | |
| **Position:** How will you position yourself for success? | |
| **Do:** Describe the transition process you expect to go through and how you'll manage it. | |

(2) Advanced Topics (going beyond the 80/20): Research "behavioral economics" to understand the psychology of rational decision-making and its impact on adopting change. It's fascinating how our mind works!

# Mark's Example

① List one change you want to make—big or small—and detail your change adoption strategy. Then, make it happen!

| | |
|---|---|
| **The Change:** Describe the change you would like to make. | *I want to significantly reduce my time watching the news and engaging in social media.* |
| **Why?:** Why would you like to make the change? | *It takes time away from more productive activities, like writing, exercising, and meditating. It also makes me unhappy as I think about the mean-spiritedness in politics and the negativity in current events. Improving in this area will significantly lift my life satisfaction.* |
| **Define:** Define what success looks like. | *A limit of 15 minutes daily spent on news and social media—just enough to stay informed. And, of course, don't get worked up!* |
| **Position:** How will you position yourself for success? | *- Set a schedule: 15 minutes in the morning.*<br><br>*- Delete news apps from my phone.*<br><br>*- Track a streak on a calendar.* |
| **Do:** Describe the transition process you expect to go through and how you'll manage it. | *I don't expect this to be a hard transition. I think making news and social media less accessible and increasing my awareness of my intention (tracking a streak) should do the trick.* |

# The Spirit

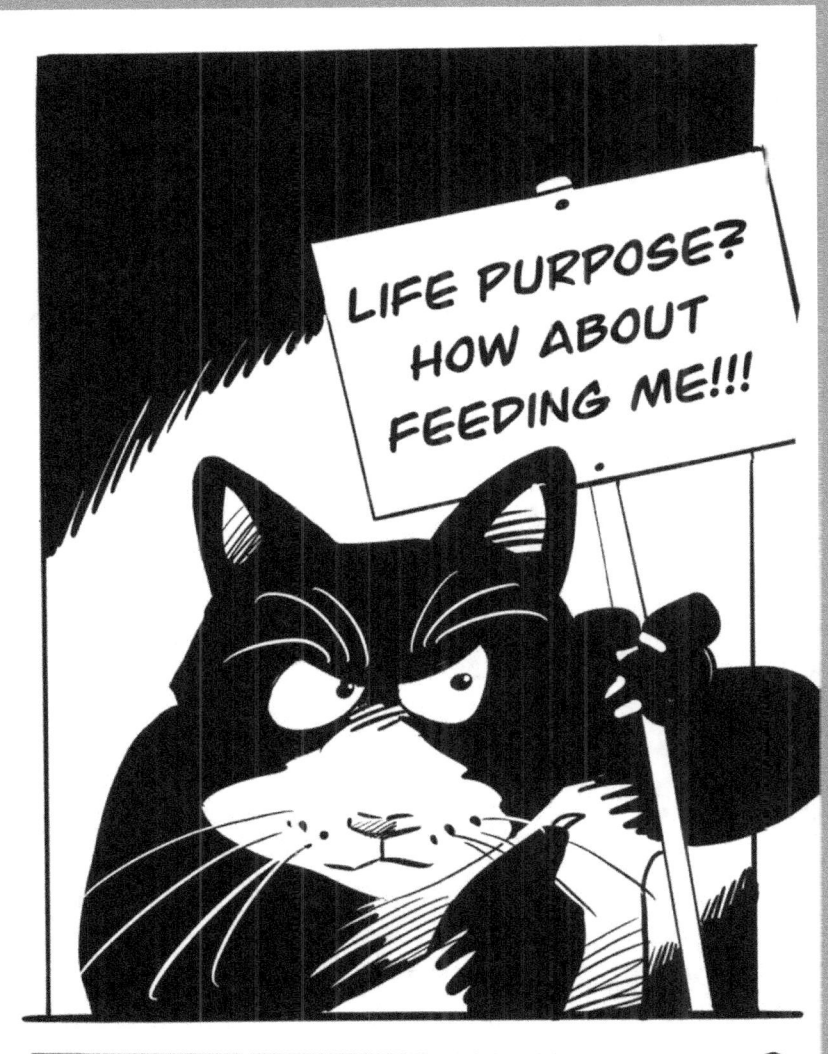

# CHAPTER 7

# A Story of Purpose

*I exist to improve people's lives through my spirit to serve, creativity, sense of humor, and ability to simplify the complex.*

That's my purpose in life, the essence of me. When your life follows the path of a noble purpose, love is created. Nothing illustrates that point better in my life than being a parent.

My parenting journey began with me being hopelessly confused. Did the "+" indicator on the home pregnancy test mean Kristen was pregnant? A reasonable person would think so, but maybe the "+" meant that my status quo wouldn't be disrupted and she wasn't pregnant. Some people would view that as a plus. I read and reread the instructions before I accepted that I was probably overthinking things.

My impending fatherhood didn't fully sink in throughout Kristen's pregnancy. But I was smart enough to know I should follow my wife's lead. So we prepped a bedroom, attended regular checkups, read *What to Expect When You're Expecting*, and childproofed our apartment.

When it came time to choose a name, I was all over that. I love naming things. I'm quite good at it. And I like to share my gift with the world. For instance, when I find out that someone I know is expecting, I'll selflessly offer to name their child for them. Inexplicably, no one has ever taken me up on that generosity, which is too bad—their offspring would have liked their names better if they had, and the world would be filled with more suitably named children. At least Kristen agreed to my proposed name for our first child: Audrey Elisabeth Reinisch.

I know it's cliché to say witnessing the birth of my child was a surreal experience, but that's the best way to describe it. During Audrey's delivery, it was like I was transported to the streets of Pamplona during the Running of the Bulls. As Kristen labored through labor, I stood attentively to the side to avoid being trampled by the devoted medical professionals. I was also careful not to draw the ire of my suffering wife by asking the staff if they had a chair I could sit on.

I remember thinking: *What does this all mean?* I was in a delivery room wearing scrubs. My wife was bravely going through childbirth as I stood there in wonderment—I was about to become a father! Was I ready to live up to that sacred responsibility?

After Audrey was born, it was a beautiful moment to see Kristen hold her for the first time. When it was my turn, I was nervous. Audrey seemed so fragile. When I held her, it finally registered—I now shared the role of raising her with my wife. It was overwhelming.

The sheer enormity of what lay ahead was beyond my understanding, so I surrendered to the unknown and went with the flow. Sometimes that's all you can do when you're tossed into a whirlwind of the daunting and unfamiliar. You enter the arena and engage like thousands have before you, if not millions or billions, depending on your endeavor. Maybe you feel like an impostor at first, but that feeling dissipates soon enough once you realize your new world isn't a pantheon inhabited by gods with mystical powers. Instead, it's a place occupied by a bunch of ordinary dolts like yourself, all at different stages in their lives and doing their best to make things work with what they've got.

I'll be vulnerable, though. I struggled at first to hit my stride as a father. I provided for Audrey and did my best to support her and Kristen. But how do I relate to a newborn? It wasn't natural for me. But soon enough, the intersection of my love for Audrey and my life purpose provided the guidance I needed.

My life purpose was unknown to my conscious mind when I was raising Audrey, but my SAGe knew it intimately and how it related to her: *I existed to improve Audrey's life through my spirit to serve, creativity, sense of humor, and ability to simplify the complex.* I intuitively embraced that role. Here are a few examples of how I lived my life purpose by being Audrey's father:

*By playing lots and lots of soccer.* Audrey dreamed of playing soccer for her high school team, even though she took up the sport a couple of years after her friends and her skills were behind. So when she was in grade school, I helped her break down where she needed to improve, and we developed drills to target those areas. We practiced for years. She ended up making the team. Nothing has been more gratifying than helping my children pursue their passions. But they always had the vision and did the work.

*By playing lots and lots of dolls.* I would play with Audrey for around ten minutes and then initiate a fight between the plastic humanoids over some perceived slight inflicted by Audrey's mean doll. Things would escalate quickly. My doll would kick Audrey's doll. Then a few body slams would occur, and maybe even some hair-pulling if my doll was really annoyed. All of this would be followed by Audrey lecturing me about proper doll-playing etiquette, and then we'd share a few laughs. Dolls are fun. I hope I have grandchildren.

*By introducing her to challenging books.* I encouraged Audrey to read for the simple joy of it, but I also influenced her to read books about subjects that might not have crossed her path otherwise, such as emotional intelligence and universal spirituality. I was delighted when she took her passion for books to another level by writing a fantasy novel during high school—I enjoyed coaching her on creative writing. I wasn't delighted when she obliterated my verbal SAT score. That was uncalled for.

I could go on—every parent has endless stories about their children. It's fascinating how life unfolds. When I think back to my experience in the delivery room, I now realize it was unreasonable for me to expect to have answers to the question: *What does this all mean?*

How could I have known what path fatherhood would lead me down, the diverse experiences I would have, and how being a father would transform my life? Or what it would feel like to see Audrey walk across a stage to receive her high school and college diplomas as tears filled my eyes? Or the pride I would feel knowing that she grew up to become an independent, super-smart, kind-hearted adult with the world at her feet?

But let me try to answer that question today by putting it through the Wellness Ethic lens.

*What does this all mean?*

The wisdom of my years tells me that the universe led me to that delivery room. To live my life purpose to its fullest potential, my journey needed to take me down the path of being a father. That's not the prescribed journey for everyone, but it was for me. I hope my children think I rose to the occasion.

*What does this all mean?*

After being in the parenting arena for nearly thirty years, here is what fatherhood means to me: I will always be there for my children in whatever capacity they need. I will do my imperfect best to teach life skills. I will serve *their* dreams and nudge them to move forward with passion, confidence, and resilience. I will coach them on how to deal with the stupid things that can happen in an unpredictable world. I will also make my fair share of well-intentioned mistakes.

Fatherhood means I will enjoy my children's company, have fun with them, celebrate their successes, and influence their sense of humor (sorry, world). I will motivate them when necessary and sometimes even inspire them. I will protect them while intentionally nurturing their independence. I will live my life purpose in ways that no other aspect of my life can match. I will become an infinitely better person by being in the parenting arena and embracing the mind-blowing responsibility.

Yes, fatherhood means far more to me than I could have imagined as a clueless, bumbling fool in his mid-twenties. And I'm curious to see how my role as a father evolves moving forward. What a life-defining blessing fatherhood has been. It has allowed me to nurture the wonderful gift of my existence.

*What does this all mean?*

Love.

o o o

# CHAPTER 8

# You Don't Need a Chatbot to Discover the Meaning of Life

When I decided to write a book about wellness, covering mind, body, spirit, and other components, I knew the spirit chapter was rife with the potential for controversy. Hell, wars have been fought throughout the ages over people's differing beliefs about God. Even today, religious intolerance fuels prejudice and violence despite the progress of human rights. This occurs with little regard for the moral incongruency inherent in inflicting emotional or physical harm on another person in the name of God.

I realize I may have offended some of my readers with that last sentence. Therein lies the difficulty in writing about the spirit. I could sidestep controversy and write a pedestrian chapter about spirituality—like a fast-food restaurant that tones down the spice to appeal to the masses—but that would be cowardly. Instead, I will authentically provide my 80/20 take and focus primarily on universal spiritual principles rather than religious dogma. At the end of this chapter, I will briefly touch upon faith and its role in spirituality.

Religion and spirituality share many similarities, but they also diverge. Religions typically approach the spiritual with defined rituals, doctrines, and institutions that prescribe a person's connection to God and a righteous order of living. Spirituality reflects a person's journey of self-discovery as they determine the meaning of their existence and how they relate to the world. It involves a transcendent feeling that there is something greater than us, that all life is connected to a higher consciousness grounded in love.

# A Level Set on the "Spirit" and Spirituality

People are sometimes confounded when they think about the meaning of the spirit. Do you have a spirit if you don't believe in God? Where did your spirit come from? What happens to it when you die? Before we explore spirituality, it's helpful to understand how the Wellness Ethic views the spirit:

*Your spirit represents the nonphysical essence of who you are.* Your life force. Your dreams and desires. Your values and humanity. Your intuition. Your spirit is what makes you uniquely *you*. When you think about the spirit in these figurative, non-ethereal terms, everyone has a "spirit" and is spiritual to some degree. The Wellness Ethic adheres to that basic notion and defines spirituality in nonreligious terms. Believing in a religion or faith has the potential to enhance a person's spirituality, but it is not required to be spiritual.

*Your spirit is naturally good.* A person's spirit is loving. It is always present and waiting to be a force of good, though it may need to be awakened sometimes. When a person does something bad, it's not because their spirit is wicked or spiteful at the core. Instead, they lost their way somehow.

*Your spirit exists on this planet for a reason.* It is important that you discover that reason—your life purpose—and align your world accordingly. You are fulfilled when the way you live honors your life purpose.

*Your spirit is different from your mind and body.* Your mind is your consciousness that controls your thoughts, actions, and emotions. Your body is your physical being. Your spirit transcends mind and body; it is your essence, your loving energy that connects you with the universe.

*Your spirit is a life partner with your mind and body.* All three work together to stabilize your earthly life. If one is out of sync with the others, dissonance occurs, and your life's positive energy flow will be stunted.

*How your spirit originated and what happens to it after death are aspects of faith.* You can still be spiritual without having answers to those questions.

We'll broaden our perspective by considering universal spirituality, representing how our spirit manifests within us and the world.

## Universal Spirituality

Calling anything "universal" can be a bold move (with universal pipe fittings being one notable exception). Proclaiming universality suggests that whatever follows the word "universal" represents the truth and is inclusive of all conditions. Such is the case with universal spirituality. But I'll take the boldness further: I believe that adopting the universal spirituality principles I'm about to share is the *most effective way* to nurture the wonderful gift of your existence, whether you follow a religion or embrace other spiritual (or nonspiritual) beliefs. But you'll draw your own conclusions—a SAGe embraces the truth that harmonizes with their benevolent spirit.

I'm wondering: Do you feel the excitement in the air, like something special is about to be revealed? Maybe even in model form if you're lucky? You have learned my ways! In keeping with my beloved 80/20 rule, the Wellness Ethic simplifies universal spirituality into three concepts: *embrace your life purpose, love the universe of existence,* and *surrender to the ways of the universe.*

### Wellness Ethic Universal Spirituality

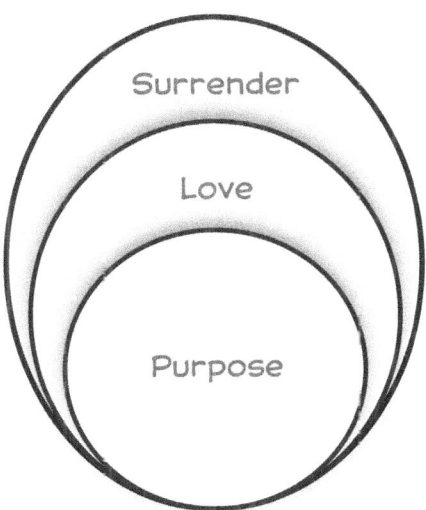

Think about what your life would be like if you fully embraced your *life purpose* and moved in that inspiring direction. Then, as you went about your day, you felt genuine *love* for all living things, including yourself, and that love was reflected in your actions and the good you propagated in the world. When stupid things occurred that you couldn't control, you chose to *surrender* to that reality and respond with your SAGe to move forward in a positive direction. A life like that would be exquisite. Maybe that already describes you.

A spiritual existence helps you realize the meaning of your life, to feel and share love. Let's unpack the model.

## Embrace Your Life Purpose

A person's life always has a purpose. That doesn't mean everyone has discovered their purpose or aligned their life accordingly. But one's life purpose is always present, either on the sidelines waiting to be thrust into the arena or as a vibrant part of one's life.

> *The two most important days in your life are the day you are born and the day you find out why.*
> —Mark Twain, American writer and humorist

I usually don't correct Mark Twain because, well, he's an American legend, and I'm told my application to become a legend was lost in the mail. Yet I will maintain that Mr. Twain should have expanded upon his quote to convey a more motivating message, something like, "The two most important days in your life are the day you are born and the day you find out why. But who gives a flyin' hoot if you don't pull up your bootstraps and do somethin' about it!"

When you understand why you were born into this world—your life purpose—and align your life accordingly, you find meaning in what you do. Work no longer feels like "work"—it's a vehicle to express the love inside of you. In your personal life, you seek experiences that manifest love. Purpose becomes the nourishment that fuels your burning desire to positively impact yourself and your world through your love-centered actions.

When you are purpose-driven, you lean into your day with an intrinsic motivation that propels you forward in alignment with your vision of a satisfying life. Purpose fosters passion, confidence, and resilience, which are essential to realizing the promise of your life.

Your life doesn't have to be world-shaking to live it on purpose. Do what you were put on this planet to do, and your life will fall into place. You'll realize its meaning, to feel and share love. You'll be amazed at the success you achieve, which, in Thoreau's words, is "unexpected in common hours."

Life purposes come in all shapes and sizes. For instance, I graduated from Beekmantown High School in 1987. Beekmantown is a rural town on the outskirts of Plattsburgh, New York, around twenty miles from the Canadian border. Graduating classes were about a hundred and fifty students. Back in 1987, the internet didn't exist in the public domain yet. Most of us didn't travel much. It was challenging to envision a world beyond the confines of our surroundings. But don't feel sorry for us; we figured out our purpose.

Today, when I look at what my former high school classmates are up to, I see them devoted to their friends and families and volunteering to make their part of the world better. I see them serving others as doctors, professors, farmers, parents, teachers, veterinarians, school administrators, psychologists, coaches, entrepreneurs, accountants, editors, business leaders, lawyers, engineers, and almost every other imaginable profession. I am heartened when I think about how a small group of Beekmantown students has impacted the world by living purposeful lives.

Every community has a similar story. This makes me optimistic about humanity's future, which, ironically, will depend upon how much humanity we bring to our everyday lives and the humanity our leaders bring to the monumental challenges we face across the globe. But don't get me started on that last one unless you want me to go on a fifty-page tirade!

To discover your life purpose, you must be in touch with who you are. What are your values? What are you really good at (your superpowers)? What do you love? The thread connecting the answers to those questions will lead you to your purpose—what you were meant to do in your life to generate love.

I'll expand upon those life purpose inputs—values, superpowers, what you love—and then, at the end of this chapter, we'll work through an exercise to personalize them, leading to crafting a life purpose statement.

## Life Purpose Input #1: Your Values

The values you hold are the ideals that define your character and guide your conduct. What fundamental beliefs are core to your Self-Actualized Genius? Not what you think society expects, but what you feel in your heart. Your values could include sacrifice, integrity, accountability, compassion, balance, humility, resilience, equality, loyalty, freedom, and more.

When you identify your values, you gain insight into the principles that shape your beliefs and priorities. This awareness leads to a better understanding of your life purpose since your life purpose is an expression of your values.

It can get tricky when you examine your values. You may find that some are not rooted in love, such as seeking revenge or winning at all costs. But those are examples of false values and are counterproductive to a spiritual life. A value must be a force of good to be spiritually authentic.

You may also find that some of your values conflict. If you value adventure and health and want to go backcountry skiing, which value wins out? Or you could compromise and find a way to honor both values by taking avalanche safety classes, avoiding high-risk terrain, and skiing with a group. Few things in life are black-and-white. Often, you need to operate in the gray and adapt your responses to serve multiple priorities.

Understanding your values and aligning your life with them is essential to realizing your spiritual potential. When you live a life misaligned with your values—valuing integrity but having an affair, valuing health but drinking to excess—you'll feel negative emotions like guilt, worry, fear, or shame. If you have compromised your values, accept and frame the spiritual disconnect, and then respond by closing the gap between your SAGe and your actions.

## Life Purpose Input #2: Your Superpowers

Everyone has genius within them. Everyone has things that they excel at. Everyone has superpowers. If someone has told you that you're not talented, I apologize on their behalf for being so shockingly ignorant. A person's superpowers could be used regularly in life, or they may have atrophied over time. They may even be undiscovered and waiting to be activated.

Typically, when you utilize your superpowers, you are fulfilled, and your self-esteem rises. You are doing what you were created to do.

To give an example of a superpower in action, my wife and I use a contractor to do various jobs around our house. It could be building a custom closet, installing lights and flooring, or anything from hundreds of projects he could skillfully complete.

His home improvement superpower is impressive. He once installed a storm door for us. It took him about forty-five minutes. He zipped through the project; the door still works perfectly.

To offer a contrast, I've also installed a storm door in the past. It took me a couple of weekends to complete the project, including fixing the many boneheaded defects in my installation. I muttered salty words that an inner-peace-loving guy like me shouldn't even know. My hammer may also have been thrown into the yard a couple of times in frustration, but I honestly don't remember if I did that during the storm door project or when I tried to build a desk—my home improvement debacles tend to conflate. I clearly don't possess the home improvement superpower, but my contractor does in a big way.

To identify your superpowers, think about what you have excelled at in your life, both personally and professionally, even during your childhood. If you asked a family member or a friend, what would they suggest? Your superpowers could include caregiving, learning languages, sports, mechanics, analytics, intelligence, writing, programming, problem-solving, building things, creativity, leadership, and others.

Thinking about your superpowers is inspiring. It opens your mind to the limitless possibilities of what you can accomplish and the love you can create when you apply your considerable talents.

## Life Purpose Input #3: What You Love

Another way to connect with your life purpose is to think about what you love. When you live your life on purpose, you manifest love. That is why purpose is so important. To get underneath what you love, consider *ordered love.*

I was first exposed to the concept of ordered love in David Brooks's book *The Road to Character.* Ordered love refers to prioritizing the things we love in our lives according to their authentic value and moral significance.[1] When you think about your career, security, family, friends, health, adventure, spirituality, giving back, integrity, and other life priorities, how would you rank them in terms of what you love the most?

Aligning your priorities with your ordered loves is integral to living a satisfying life. If you prioritize a lower love over a higher love, you create a disconnect that can undermine your spirit. Do you have health and family at the top of your list of loves but allow your job to dominate your life? Or do you compromise your integrity for material gain, even when integrity is a higher love? If the priorities in your life feel out of sync, choose your SAGe-inspired response to better align your life with what you love the most.

Now that we have a wealth of inputs, the next step is to craft a life purpose statement that will answer the spiritual question: How can I realize the meaning of my life (to feel and share love)? Your life purpose statement will help you define your very existence. No pressure.

## Crafting Your Life Purpose Statement

A life purpose statement—your *why*—reflects how you want to live your life to manifest love and impact the world. The statement should align with your values, superpowers, and loves, and it should inspire you. It doesn't have to alter the course of history. It can reflect the influence you want to have in your community, with your family, or even on yourself—choose a level of impact that will fulfill you.

A good litmus test for whether your life purpose statement captures your true why is envisioning being on your deathbed and looking back at your life. At that moment of truth, if you had lived your purpose throughout your days, would you be satisfied with your life? Would you have released the love inside of you? If so, your life purpose represents why you were born into this world. If not, then you have more reflection to do.

Though there is no standard format for a life purpose statement—you should use the style and format that resonates—I'll offer a simple framework to get your mind thinking about your purpose:

### Life Purpose Statement
**I [what you do to impact the world] through my [how you do it].**

Your values, superpowers, and loves inform what you do and how you do it. Here are examples of life purpose statements utilizing the framework:

○ I exist to help young people realize their potential through my empathy, wisdom, and mentoring.

○ I free animals from suffering through my compassion and activism.

○ I was born to make the world beautiful through my artistic talents.

○ I bring justice to those in need through my advocacy and legal acumen.

○ I am devoted to saving our planet for future generations by doing my part and leading others to do the same.

○ I inspire the world to grow spiritually through my gift of storytelling.

You may have noticed that these life purpose statements don't detail exactly what a person does to achieve their purpose; instead, they provide a theme for one's life. They point in a direction mainly in the person's control. The statements recognize that there are many ways to live a life on purpose.

Consider the life purpose statement: "I exist to help young people realize their potential through my empathy, wisdom, and mentoring." It sounds like the life purpose statement of a teacher, right? It could be. But it also could describe a parent, a daycare provider, a mentor, a community volunteer, a youth minister, a coach, a philanthropist, and hundreds of other endeavors. There is never just one path leading you to the promised land of a fulfilling, purpose-driven life—there are many. And if you don't see a path, rent a bulldozer and clear your own.

By keeping your life purpose statement at the thematic level, you'll give yourself ample room to explore your purpose in diverse and inspired ways.

Throughout the rest of this book, I encourage you to put all aspects of your life through the life purpose lens. How can your mind, body, and spirit support your life purpose? How can your relationships and personal and professional pursuits help you feel and share love? What about lifestyle maintenance?

Aligning the important aspects of your life with your purpose is a way to supercharge your existence. It's like a close-knit volleyball team working together seamlessly on the court as they compete for a championship.

## Love the Universe of Existence

Love is the meaning of your life. It is the why behind your purpose, the reason why you exist. A life without love is the equivalent of hiking in the Grand Tetons with your head down, glued to your phone as you tune out Mother Nature's splendor (and probably bump into an angry moose as a result).

Love is the common denominator that connects all living things. A devotion to love will make you happier, less stressed, and more fulfilled. You'll attract positivity into your life, whether it's through more opportunities, richer experiences, or deeper relationships. You won't get worked up by life's bloated dramas. I could go on, but you get it—**love is everything!**

When you *love the universe of existence*, you feel and share love. Your life force is filled to the brim with affection, care, and connection. Love is your default setting when you wake up in the morning, and you nurture love throughout the day. When you love the universe of existence, you:

- love yourself.
- appreciate your Mona Lisa moments.
- lead with love.
- practice radical gratitude.
- purge the dispiriting virus from your life.
- feel connected to the universe of existence.

You know the routine by now. We'll dive off the deep end and start swimming in the details, beginning with *love yourself.*

## Love Yourself

Love starts and ends with you. In between is the love you share with others. When you love yourself, you embrace your spiritual essence as good. You know you have a lot to offer the world. You believe that you deserve happiness and fulfillment, and you move your life in a direction that realizes that promise. You enjoy your successes, savor your life, and cut yourself slack when you struggle because you know everyone is a perpetual work in progress. You accept your appearance as perfectly you, no matter what others may say. When you love yourself, every cell in your body knows that you matter.

When your life force isn't strengthened by self-love, you may be happy sometimes, but it will be short-lived. Invariably, dissatisfaction with your *perception* of who you are and the state of your life will surface, wrecking your equilibrium.

Loving yourself *less* may be triggered by an unfulfilled dream, seeing a colleague get a promotion and erroneously thinking they're more successful than you, wishing there was something different about your appearance, or a breakup with a partner. Just about anything can become an invalid reason for someone to love themselves less. Sidestep the love-diminishing traps always present and accept the indisputable truth: **You are worthy of love.**

If you are challenged in this area, loop back to the previous chapters on choosing your response to life and adopting change. What techniques can you use to boost your self-love? Here are five ideas: (1) Choose to practice self-compassion by treating yourself to the kindness you would offer a friend in need. (2) Create positive affirmations and develop a daily habit of repeating them, such as "I am worthy of love and respect" and "I have a lot of love to offer to myself and the world." (3) Go through a 5 Whys exercise to get underneath your limiting beliefs about your perceived unworthiness of love. Develop a change adoption plan to shift your mindset. (4) Make it a daily habit to do something that brings you joy. Maintain the streak for the rest of your life. (5) Seek professional help if you struggle to feel good about yourself.

## Appreciate Your Mona Lisa Moments

When I saw the *Mona Lisa* in person years ago at the Louvre, I was taken aback by the alluring beauty of Leonardo da Vinci's painting. There had been so much hype about the masterpiece that I almost expected it to be a tourist trap—you see the artwork, check the box that you saw it, take the obligatory selfie, and then move on. But that wasn't my experience. Like millions before me, I was mesmerized by the mystery of her expression and how she flowed seamlessly into the distant countryside. I thought about Leonardo's Renaissance genius and was thrilled to experience his immortal gift firsthand.

As I think about my enchanting visit to the Louvre, I'm struck by the notion that I encounter at least a dozen Mona Lisa moments each day *if I'm open to such experiences.* They're experiences that can entrance my senses, fill my heart with love, and make me appreciate being alive. Let me share some examples of my everyday Mona Lisa moments so you can see what I mean:

○ My wife and I live in a house with a wooded backyard. A stray cat, whom I named Christopher McFluffer (he looked like a McFluffer), appeared one day and demanded that we become his caregiver. He wasn't willing to negotiate. So we feed him every morning and evening. We have no choice—he'll stare at us through our windows with needy eyes until we do so. He now hangs out on ~~our~~ his stone patio throughout the day, basking in the sun, safe from predators. If we travel overnight, we arrange for a cat sitter to tend to him. We're lucky to have an opportunity to make a difference in the life of a stray cat. It brings us joy. Here's a picture of the peeping McFluffer:

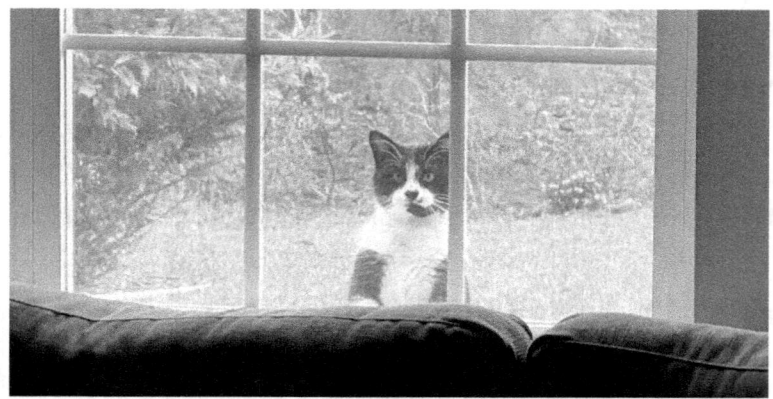

○ When my wife and I moved to South Carolina, we visited art galleries in downtown Charleston. It was a sensory explosion that hooked me. I've been fortunate to purchase several paintings from gifted artists. Each day, the paintings fill my spirit with inspiration.

○ During my early morning walks around my neighborhood, depending upon the time I leave, I may experience a gorgeous sunrise, deer stampeding in front of me, a full moon illuminating the night, terrified toads hopping out of the way of my duck-like feet, or even a water moccasin on a sidewalk daring me to come just a wee bit closer. I love nature, except nature that injects venom into human bloodstreams.

Each moment in your life can be a Mona Lisa moment if you appreciate what the universe offers you and mindfully engage your senses. Doing so helps you feel love in the present. What are your Mona Lisa moments?

## Lead with Love

You think differently when you put your experiences through the lens of love *before* passing judgment. You think more clearly and in harmony with your spirit's inherent goodness. Your SAGe becomes inspired to choose a life-affirming frame that helps you maintain your optimism.

When you take it a step further and choose the most loving response possible to a situation, you produce love within yourself and the world. That's leading with love's ultimate objective—create as much love as possible from your experiences. If people (politicians, business leaders, you, me, everyone) led with love, our world would be profoundly different. We would be happier. Our relationships would thrive. The world would cooperate to end hunger and address climate change. War wouldn't exist. There wouldn't be inequality. Imagine what the world would be like if love guided our collective actions.

Let's take *lead with love* for a test drive: Your flight has been canceled due to a tropical storm, and you are waiting in a long line to book another flight.

You have a choice in how you'll handle the situation, whether you'll lead with love or not. You have no control over the flight cancellation (nor does anyone else), but you could choose to be angry, which would raise your blood pressure and probably give you a headache. You could share your frustration with everyone around you, which will suck positive energy from them.

When you reach the beleaguered ticketing agent, you could tell them exactly how you feel, blaming them for their mortal inability to manipulate the weather. You may even choose to spew colorful vulgarities just in case anyone doubts how much contempt you feel toward the reality that something happened in your life that you couldn't control! Would any of those unloving responses serve you or anyone in a positive way?

Or you could choose to lead with love. You could surrender to what happened and accept that it is out of your control. You would be happier as a result. You could be pleasant to those around you and even more pleasant to the stressed-out ticketing agent. It would probably make everyone's day. By leading with love, you would still get your flight rescheduled, and you would have created positive energy in the universe.

When you lead with love, you lead with empathy and care. You recognize that everyone has stuff going on in their lives that you're not privy to. You realize that everyone is imperfect and deserves a break. You believe that everyone deserves love, including yourself. You choose a love-centered response to life that creates the best outcomes for everyone involved.

Here's another reason to lead with love. When you lead with love and impact the lives of others, a miraculous thing happens: Not only do you lift their lives, but you also bring more love into your life. When you share love, you feel love. It's how love works. It's kind of cool.

Are you willing to lead with love to make our shared world better? I've signed up for that, unless I encounter a water moccasin.

## Practice Radical Gratitude

We all want more. It's okay to admit it. For example, if you joyfully devour a mouthwatering piece of huckleberry pie that reaffirms that pie is vastly superior to cake (you know I'm right), you probably would like another slice. If you make more money than you need, you wouldn't mind a 10% raise. And if you rise to that higher salary, you'll soon set your sights on earning more. It's human nature to normalize around your lot in life, and then want more.

A SAGe may *want* more in their life, whether it's finding more inner peace, having more financial security, or experiencing more adventure. But the SAGe is radically grateful for the blessings they already have and believes they don't really *need* anything else to be satisfied.

When you practice radical gratitude, you mindfully and spiritually connect with the good in your life that has always been present—you just needed to engage with it. You appreciate your blessings—both big and small—and embrace the love in your relationships. You savor experiences and find silver linings in adversity. You have a generous spirit.

Looking at my life, I could dwell on my unfulfilled desires to live in a large lake house, have more time to pursue my writing passion, and buy expensive art I can't afford. I could get frustrated with my dryer breaking down, the incessant demands of my job, and the many mistakes I've made in the past. That's a dump-truckload of dissatisfaction I could welcome into my life.

Or I could be radically grateful that I'm blessed with a wonderful family. I could be radically grateful that my wife and I live in a comfortable house that meets our needs, and I have a job that provides the income to cover life's necessities. I have many blessings that may seem like entitlements but are not—they're not guaranteed to be a part of my life. When I radically appreciate the gift of what I have rather than dwelling on what I don't have, I realize I already have everything I need.

What are the blessings in your life? Take a moment and list them. Then, radically appreciate the gift of the universe's blessings and emotionally connect with the love you feel. You can also consider creating a gratitude journal to capture your list and establishing a habit of adding to it (and reviewing it) regularly. It will lift your spirits. It may even transform your mindset.

## Purge the Dispiriting Virus from Your Life

It takes conditioning not to love. When a child is born, they don't feel prejudice or hatred. A child is trusting and curious. They feel a natural affinity toward others. But over time, they are introduced to inequality, bullying, violence, hate, injustice, and other spiritual counterforces that erode their love-centered mindset.

As the child matures into adulthood, their spirit will have become infected, to some degree, with a dispiriting virus that feeds on the constant barrage of negative reinforcement in their environment. Left untreated, the virus multiplies and can further sap their capacity to love.

I understand that what I'm about to share may be a humbling jolt to your sensibilities, but here it goes: We have all been infected by a dispiriting virus. No matter how spiritual you are or how much love you feel in your heart, you are human. You can't help but be impacted by negative forces around you. You may be cynical, jaded, or withdrawn on occasion. You may feel angry at times. Or violence, hate, dishonesty, self-dealing, or other character-suffocating energies may have overtaken your life.

Wherever you're at, the dispiriting virus is constantly wrestling with your SAGe for control of you. The dispiriting virus wants you to live in the depths of despair. After all, misery loves company. When you love the universe of existence—when your life force is saturated with love—you choose better company, and your life takes off in wonderful and unexpected ways.

To purge the dispiriting virus from your life, you can start by assessing which influences have spread negativity throughout your mind and spirit. Here are some common culprits:

- Cable news and social media that promote conspiracies and division

- Friends, family, or work colleagues who bring negativity into your life

- Working at a company with a corrosive culture

- Your actions that run counter to your spiritual values

- The state of the world: climate change, war, famine, oppression

- A grudge that you hold

Once you have pinpointed a source of negativity, work through the Accept-Frame-Respond model to choose a spiritual response to bring love into your life. Do you need to let go of something that happened in the past? Or make a career change? Do you need to shift the dynamics in a relationship? Wherever your opportunities lie, ask yourself: Am I willing to cede control of my happiness to an outside force or my self-sabotaging behavior?

## Feel Connected to the Universe of Existence

What is your frame of reference when you think about your place in the universe? Do you see yourself as an individual who is independent of others?

Do you view yourself as a member of a tribe, and that forms your identity? Or, and this is provocative, do you envision yourself connected to all living things, an interdependent collective consciousness?

When you feel connected to the universe of existence, you recognize that you are an integral part of a greater whole. You love life, care for all living things, and strive to alleviate suffering. You understand that life isn't just about you; there's a bigger picture centered around creating harmony with humanity and nature to propagate love in the universe.

Consider what Alan Shepard, a NASA astronaut, thought after gazing at Earth from space: "I realized up there that our planet is not infinite. It's fragile. That may not be obvious to a lot of folks, and it's tough that people are fighting each other here on Earth instead of trying to get together and live on this planet. We look pretty vulnerable in the darkness of space."

When you're woven into the fabric of the universe of existence, you connect with the beauty of the mysterious, interconnected ecosystem whose inhabitants must love one another to survive. In this grander scheme, your life matters. Yet you are one human among billions. You are one human among trillions of other life forms, ranging from the smallest amoeba to the tallest redwood. Does that humble you? It should.

To feel connected to the universe of existence, a starting point can be to connect more deeply with the love in your relationships. Feel a sense of empathy, affection, and unity toward those who are in your orbit. Embrace each person's vibrant essence. Then, expand your loving horizons throughout the rest of the universe of existence by doing the following:

When you walk in a crowd, be an astute observer and imagine the people around you having lives filled with family, friends, and dreams. They've experienced joy and hardship. They deserve love in their life. They're just like you. Connect with their humanity. Feel love within you.

When you walk in nature, observe the birds flying. Listen to their cheerful chirps. Imagine their tiny hearts beating. See the butterfly flapping its colorful wings as it bobs in the breeze. Or a spider weaving its life-sustaining web. Every living thing has a purpose in this symbiotic ecosystem and must work together in the circle of life to thrive. Connect with that oneness. Feel love within you.

What will you do today to feel connected to the universe of existence?

## Surrender to the Ways of the Universe

You embrace your life purpose. Your life purpose is your tour guide to living a fulfilled life. You love the universe of existence. You approach each day with kindness as you bring love to yourself and others, giving Earth a bounce to its orbit. Then, life tosses a curveball and throws you off balance. That's when *surrender to the ways of the universe* enters the spiritual game and helps you pick up the spin on the ball to put it in play.

When you surrender to the ways of the universe, you choose to release the need to control the natural flow of life. You trust that events will unfold as they are intended. By accepting your lack of control over the natural order, you liberate your mind and spirit to focus on what you can always control: your thoughts and responses to life. Surrendering provides a path to inner peace.

A key aspect of surrendering to the ways of the universe is accepting that impermanence is an inescapable truth that reflects the nature of existence as it is, not necessarily as you would like it to be.

### The Law of Impermanence

Sunrise and sunset. Birth and death. Changing seasons. Evolution. These are just some examples of nature's impermanence. But look at your life's progression—employment, relationships, finances, health, where you live . . . Do you notice anything in common? Yep, more impermanence. More change. That's what the Law of Impermanence teaches us: Everything changes. Everything has a beginning, middle, and end.

Existence is synonymous with change. You can fight it and sometimes delay it, but change will march on like a determined emperor penguin heading to its breeding colony. **Change is the way of the universe.**

*Whatever has the nature of arising has the nature of ceasing.*
—The Buddha

As an example of change, consider your body—it will age and break down. Guaranteed. No human has ever escaped that fate. How long will your body be alive, and what will be your quality of life at any given moment? No one knows. Not even the most gifted data scientist, using the most sophisticated machine learning algorithms, can predict with certainty what will happen to your body, except that it will continuously change.

When you embrace the Law of Impermanence, you surrender to the truth that change is constant. That wisdom becomes an integral part of your empowering worldview, a worldview that chooses to flow with the current of change rather than trying to paddle upstream to reach a past-tense reality that is no longer there. You act like a dogwood tree that surrenders to winter by shedding its leaves and preserving energy so it can blossom in the spring.

For a Self-Actualized Genius, surrendering to impermanence can mean:

○ *As the SAGe grows older, they may fondly reflect upon their youth, but they accept their advancing age as unavoidable. They find joy and meaning in the present and evolve their life based on their reality.*

○ *When a loved one passes away, the SAGe understands and accepts that life has a beginning, middle, and end.* They grieve, for that is a loving and natural response, but they emerge grateful for their loved one's time on earth as they move forward in their own life. Their suffering recedes as a result.

○ *As relationships evolve in a SAGe's life, the SAGe evolves with them.* The SAGe recognizes that the most meaningful relationship is between two people who keep their love flourishing as they grow throughout their unique but overlapping life journeys. The SAGe also acknowledges that some relationships run their natural course and go dormant. That can be okay, too, if that's what is meant to be.

○ *When the SAGe experiences something positive, they are grateful for their blessing but understand that their status quo is not permanent.* Therefore, they are careful to moderate their attachment to what they have today because they know it will change tomorrow.

○ *When the SAGe experiences down periods, they understand that all things pass because all things change.* This helps them shorten the suffering cycle because they know their present state is not permanent.

The Law of Impermanence, which is fundamental to many Eastern and Western spiritual traditions, encourages you to accept and frame change as inevitable, allow life to unfold naturally, and then choose your loving response to your reality to move your life forward.

*To everything there is a season, and a time to every purpose under the heaven.*
—Ecclesiastes 3:1

## I Surrender Because I Am One

*The wisp of life against the backdrop of the ages,*
*I surrender because I am humble.*

*The faithful current that ferries glorious dreams,*
*I surrender because I am on purpose.*

*The unbearable weight of a million mirages,*
*I surrender because I am unattached.*

*An encounter with circumstance that cannot be foretold,*
*I surrender because I am strong.*

*The mysterious origin of a fortuitous beginning,*
*I surrender because I am awake.*

*The mighty gale that nudges a ship to uncharted seas,*
*I surrender because I am trusting.*

*The rumbling ground beneath the chosen path,*
*I surrender because I am courageous.*

*The knowing spirit that transcends mind and body,*
*I surrender because I am wise.*

*The unyielding march of the abundant moment,*
*I surrender because I am grateful.*

*The torrential monsoon that floods the parched land,*
*I surrender because I am one.*

—Mark Reinisch

## Should You Have Faith?

Embracing your life purpose, loving the universe of existence, and surrendering to the ways of the universe are fundamentals of spiritual wellness. I would suggest they are universal beliefs that don't require a leap of faith to recognize their inherent value in promoting good in your life. But what about spiritual beliefs that do require a leap of faith? Beliefs that can't be scientifically proven, such as life after death or the existence of God? Do faith-based beliefs have a place in spirituality? They can, *if that's what you choose.*

Faith is defined as believing in something without proof. When faith is misplaced, it can be destructive. For example, if a person places their trust in harmful conspiracy theories or immoral leaders, they can belly flop their life into a toxic cesspool that drowns their spirit. **A general rule of thumb for faith is that it can be a positive force in your life if it promotes good and doesn't harm others.**

Most religions have faith-based beliefs that are core to their teachings. The beliefs vary, but prevalent themes exist, including the ideas that God created the universe and serves as the supreme being overseeing all; there is life after death; God performs miracles impacting human lives; prayer creates more favorable outcomes for those who pray; and how you conduct your life determines your fate in the afterlife.

Which faith-based beliefs should you embrace, if any? That's up to you. It's important for people to reach their own conclusions.

We exist in the universe to feel and share love. Spirituality, whether universal or faith-based, can be your best path to manifesting this magnificent promise.

○ ○ ○

## Move Forward on Your Wellness Ethic Journey!

① Complete the My Compass tool to identify your life purpose.

| My Compass | |
|---|---|
| **Values** | **Your Top 5** |
| ○ Accountability ○ Achievement ○ Adventure ○ Authenticity ○ Balance ○ Character ○ Commitment ○ Compassion & Empathy ○ Courage ○ Creativity ○ Diversity, Equity & Inclusion ○ Flexibility ○ Forgiveness ○ Freedom ○ Giving Back ○ Gratitude ○ Growth & Learning ○ Happiness ○ Health & Wellness ○ Honesty ○ Hope ○ Humility ○ Humor ○ Inspiration ○ Integrity ○ Justice ○ Kindness ○ Love ○ Loyalty ○ Meaning & Purpose ○ Optimism ○ Patience ○ Peace ○ Prosperity ○ Resilience ○ Respect ○ Sacrifice ○ Safety & Security ○ Simplicity ○ Spirituality ○ Surrender ○ Trust ○ Wisdom ○ _____ ○ _____ | |
| **Superpowers** | **Your Top 4** |
| ○ Analytics ○ Attention to Detail ○ Building Things ○ Caregiving ○ Communication ○ Conflict Resolution ○ Creativity ○ Decision-Making ○ Design ○ Emotional Intelligence ○ Engineering ○ Financial Management ○ Humor ○ Inspiration ○ Intelligence ○ Languages ○ Leadership ○ Marketing ○ Mechanics ○ Memory ○ Music ○ Negotiation ○ Networking ○ Organization ○ Problem-Solving ○ Programming ○ Research ○ Self-Control ○ Service ○ Spirituality ○ Sports ○ Strategic Thinking ○ Systems Thinking ○ Teaching ○ Teamwork ○ Technology ○ Time Management ○ Wisdom ○ Writing ○ _____ ○ _____ | |
| **Ordered Love** | **Your Top 5** |
| ○ Adventure ○ Animals ○ Art ○ Creativity ○ Family ○ Food ○ Friends ○ Giving Back ○ Health ○ Hobbies ○ Independence ○ Integrity ○ Learning ○ Leisure ○ Music ○ Nature ○ Professional Achievement ○ Reputation ○ Security ○ Spirituality ○ Sports & Recreation ○ Technology ○ _____ ○ _____ | |
| **Your Life Purpose Statement** | |
| | |

② What steps can you take to enhance how you *embrace your life purpose*, *love the universe of existence*, and *surrender to the ways of the universe*? How will you approach change adoption?

③ Is there a *faith* component to your spirituality? If so, how would you describe it?

④ Advanced Topics (going beyond the 80/20): When you feel connected to the universe of existence, you tap into spiritual energy to achieve inner peace. Consider trying other spiritual practices (beyond what was covered in this chapter) to connect with the universe, such as yoga, meditation, Reiki (a Japanese healing practice), and others.

## Mark's Example

(1) Complete the My Compass tool to identify your life purpose.

| My Compass | |
|---|---|
| **Values** | **Your Top 5** |
| o Accountability o Achievement o Adventure o Authenticity o Balance o Character o Commitment o Compassion & Empathy o Courage o Creativity o Diversity, Equity & Inclusion o Flexibility o Forgiveness o Freedom o Giving Back o Gratitude o Growth & Learning o Happiness o Health & Wellness o Honesty o Hope o Humility o Humor o Inspiration o Integrity o Justice o Kindness o Love o Loyalty o Meaning & Purpose o Optimism o Patience o Peace o Prosperity o Resilience o Respect o Sacrifice o Safety & Security o Simplicity o Spirituality o Surrender o Trust o Wisdom o _____ o _____ | - Love<br>- Integrity<br>- Meaning &<br>Purpose<br>- Creativity<br>- Surrender |
| **Superpowers** | **Your Top 4** |
| o Analytics o Attention to Detail o Building Things o Caregiving o Communication o Conflict Resolution o Creativity o Decision-Making o Design o Emotional Intelligence o Engineering o Financial Management o Humor o Inspiration o Intelligence o Languages o Leadership o Marketing o Mechanics o Memory o Music o Negotiation o Networking o Organization o Problem-Solving o Programming o Research o Self-Control o Service o Spirituality o Sports o Strategic Thinking o Systems Thinking o Teaching o Teamwork o Technology o Time Management o Wisdom o Writing o _____ o _____ | - Servant<br>Leadership<br>(Service)<br>- Creativity<br>- Strategic<br>Thinking<br>- Systems<br>Thinking |
| **Ordered Love** | **Your Top 5** |
| o Adventure o Animals o Art o Creativity o Family o Food o Friends o Giving Back o Health o Hobbies o Independence o Integrity o Learning o Leisure o Music o Nature o Professional Achievement o Reputation o Security o Spirituality o Sports & Recreation o Technology o _____ o _____ | 1. Integrity<br>2. Family<br>3. Health<br>4. Spirituality<br>5. Creativity |
| **Your Life Purpose Statement** | |
| *I exist to improve people's lives through my spirit to serve, creativity, sense of humor, and ability to simplify the complex.* | |

② What steps can you take to enhance how you *embrace your life purpose, love the universe of existence*, and *surrender to the ways of the universe*? How will you approach change adoption?

> *I will lead with love by keeping love in the forefront of my mind as I engage in life. I will choose better responses as a result. I will place a note with the word "Love" on my computer monitor as a form of visual management to keep this intention in front of me.*
>
> *I need to think through how well my profession aligns with my life purpose. There may be opportunities to do something different within my company or make a career pivot. I'm not ready to commit to a change just yet, but I will begin to consider possibilities.*

③ Is there a *faith* component to your spirituality? If so, how would you describe it?

> *The central belief in my faith is that there is a God. I don't assign a name to that God. I view God as the life force that is a part of all of us. That is why I feel connected to all living things. It also compels me to care about and serve others.*
>
> *I believe that my spirit carries on after death of my physical body. I am comforted when I think about death as another step in my spirit's journey, that more love and experiences lie ahead for me after I die.*
>
> *I believe in the power of positive thinking and have faith that positive thoughts attract positive energy.*

# The Mind

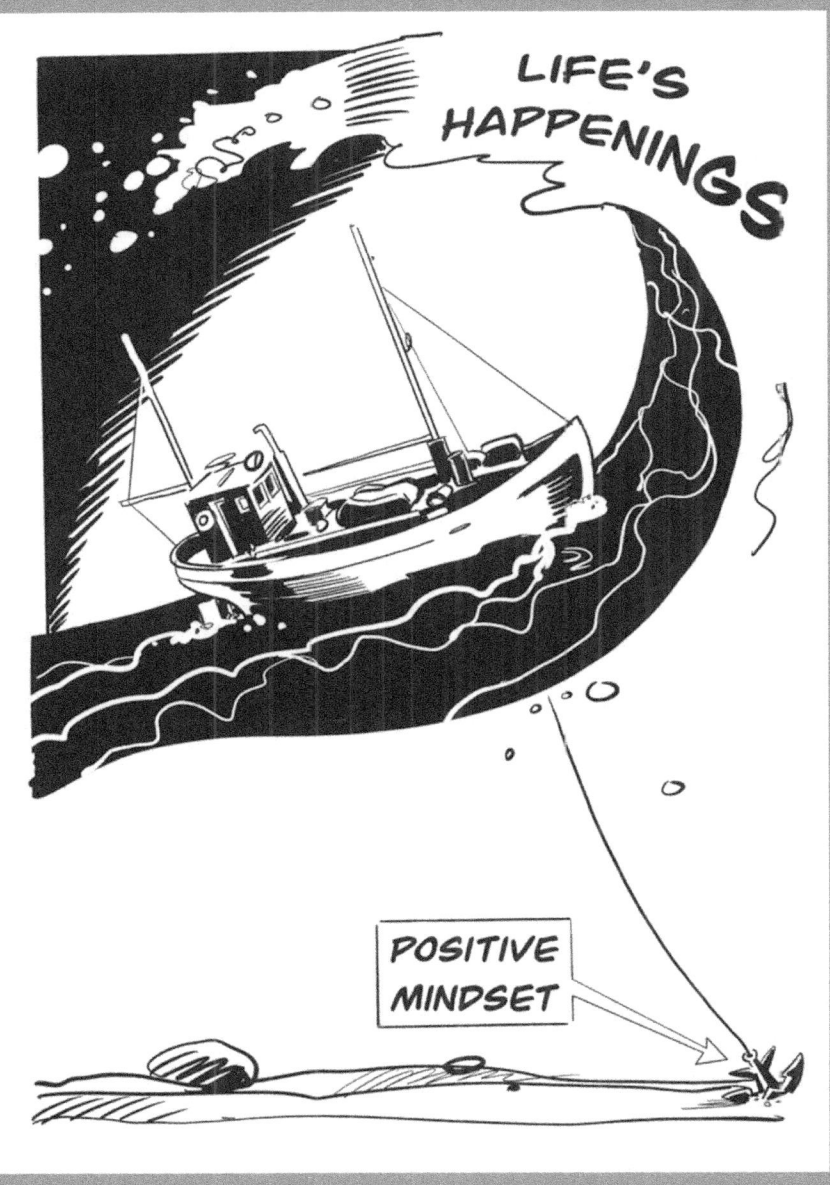

# CHAPTER 9

# A Story of Courage

"Wait, wait a second. You've had a nonstop headache for five days?" I asked my daughter Emma incredulously while we stood in our Florida kitchen with my wife, Kristen.

"Yes," Emma replied. "It started on Saturday."

"What has been the pain level, on a scale of one to ten?"

"I don't know. Maybe a five or six."

"We think it might be allergies or a sinus infection," Kristen interjected.

"That can't be it. Not for five days." I turned back to Emma. "Did anything trigger this? I mean, did you hit your head on something?"

"No. I don't know what's going on." Emma was usually five chess moves ahead of me in her thought process. She was smarter than me (by a lot), and she was only a high school sophomore. In this case, she had already processed through the potential root causes and hit a dead end.

I looked to Kristen. "Do we have a doctor's appointment set up?"

"Not yet," Kristen answered.

"We need to see a doctor urgently." I didn't want to share what was running through my über-panicked mind. The words were unspeakable.

Emma bolted from the womb in 2001. Once Kristen began to push, twenty minutes later, Emma was born. It was like she couldn't wait to start leaving her mark on this world. Growing up, Emma left no doubt that she was the producer of *The Emma Show*. For instance, when she was eight, she decided to become a vegetarian. I wasn't thrilled with that due to my ignorance of nutrition at the time, but Emma ferreted out the illogic coming from her poor, overmatched father and countered my hesitancy with facts. She won the battle of wits and never strayed from her commitment to forgo meat.

Emma was socially active in middle school. Still, she was also head-down focused on positioning herself to be accepted at her dream college, Cornell University, to study veterinary medicine. She was involved in school extracurriculars, took college-level courses in the summer as a part of Duke TIP (Talent Identification Program), and wrote fantasy novels. Emma loved challenging what was possible in her life, which thrilled me. It told me that her passion for new experiences came from her heart.

Emma was on a special path as high school loomed. Little did we know that she would soon begin an excruciating medical odyssey that would change her life forever and still overwhelm her parents' emotions to this day.

Entering high school, one of Emma's passions was rowing. She took it up in eighth grade and quickly fell in love with the physicality of sculling. She also saw the sport as an angle to get a Division I athletic scholarship, which could open the door to expensive out-of-state colleges otherwise out of reach.

Then, life threw a nasty curveball when she was accustomed to seeing fastballs down the middle. While jogging at rowing practice in the fall of her freshman year, she experienced piercing shoulder pain that stopped her in her tracks. The pain continued for a couple of weeks whenever she jogged.

Soon, the pain became constant. Kristen and I took her to an orthopedist, who diagnosed her with a torn labrum and shoulder hypermobility. The doctor also noticed that Emma's hypermobility affected all her joints throughout her body, but none of us were concerned—she had always been like that.

After months of physical therapy to no avail, major shoulder surgery was required. Emma had the surgery in March of her freshman year and endured months of painful rehab afterward. Her rowing career was over since there was a strong likelihood that the repeated motion from rowing would cause a flare-up of her shoulder issues, probably requiring further surgery.

With rowing no longer an option, Emma had to recalibrate her life. She shifted gears and planned to join the cross-country running team in the fall. I was super proud of her positive and resilient mindset when facing obstacles.

Then, another curveball was thrown her way: She broke her ankle at the end of her freshman year when she stood up from a chair. Her foot had fallen asleep, and she twisted her ankle when she started to walk. We learned afterward that it was common for her legs to fall asleep while sitting, even when they weren't crossed. The doctors viewed the shoulder and ankle issues as disconnected. The following two years would prove otherwise.

Emma's broken ankle required surgery. Cross-country running was no longer an option. In an Energizer Bunny–like fashion, Emma once again accepted her reality and chose her response to her setback. She decided to pursue competitive bike racing once her ankle recovered. We even dreamed of riding our bikes across Florida and sharing other epic biking adventures.

Emma had demonstrated a remarkably mature perspective about how life worked as she weathered a monsoon of adversity. Though she didn't like what was happening to her, she surrendered to the ways of the universe and stubbornly refused to let what she couldn't control stop her from finding ways to love the universe of existence and embrace her life purpose. She had valiantly reestablished equilibrium despite the disruptive counterforces. The headaches would soon blow up that balance with the explosive might of a thousand sticks of dynamite.

Emma's chronic daily headaches started in November of her sophomore year. She saw several neurologists and other specialists and went through a battery of tests—MRIs, blood tests, allergy tests—but nothing pointed to the root cause of her condition. The doctors had ruled out a brain tumor, which was a colossal relief, but she was miserable.

This is what she endured: Imagine having a splitting headache, to a five-to six-level (out of ten), every single minute of every single day, nonstop. Literally nonstop. Minute after minute. Day after day. Week after week. Not a measly second of reprieve in your waking hours from the onslaught of pain.

And then, as if that's not enough extreme suffering for a person to endure, at least five times a week, you get a crushing migraine headache that jacks up the pain to an eight- to ten-level, and the migraine and its prodrome and postdrome effects last for hours upon hours. You are in constant pain. You are exhausted and falling behind in school. Your life has been upended, and you have no idea what the hell is going on! Is this a permanent state? Will you live the rest of your life like this? No idea. Will things improve over time, or will your condition deteriorate further? Again, no f***ing idea!!!

To make matters worse, the medications the doctors prescribed didn't reduce the pain or headache frequency. They also had many side effects, including muddling Emma's brain and, at times, cruelly raising her pain level. Nothing was working. It was heartbreaking. It was frustrating! That's how Kristen and I felt. But imagine being Emma. I couldn't imagine being Emma.

We had settled into a routine out of necessity. Emma desperately wanted to live on *her* terms, so despite having a constant headache that would compel an ordinary person to take a sick day and rest in bed, Emma bravely chose to go to school. Unfortunately, part of the routine also included Kristen picking her up after lunch because that's when Emma's daily migraine would begin to rear its god-awful head and deliver extreme pain, nausea, and light-and-noise sensitivity.

Once Emma was home, Kristen would serve as her nurse and help her in any way she could, whether it was massaging her head, fixing her favorite food, getting an ice pack, or setting up Emma's room—close the shade, turn off the lights, turn on the fan, get another blanket, locate one of the cats to provide comfort, whatever Emma wanted.

In trying times like this, I was grateful that Kristen had decided to become a stay-at-home mom when our first child, Audrey, was a toddler. We weren't rolling in money by any stretch, but we made the financial sacrifice so Kristen could fully realize her life purpose of becoming the best mom she could be. Having a parent give up their paycheck to raise their children full-time isn't the right decision for every family—every person, every family has different considerations to balance—but it was the right decision for us.

After winter break, Emma began her spring semester. Her headaches hadn't improved. She continued to come home in the afternoon due to her migraines, making her fall further behind in school. It was clear that Emma needed to transition to virtual learning. This was pre-pandemic, so the notion of a virtual school was a paradigm shift for us. Still, all Kristen and I cared about was Emma's well-being. Emma also cared about her well-being, of course, but how she'd get there—the journey she'd embark upon—inspires me to this day. As I said, Emma was usually five chess moves ahead of me.

As Emma began homeschooling, our focus was to stabilize her life while working with her doctors to determine what was causing her headaches and how they could be treated. Emma became a clinical trial of one as she went from specialist to specialist and tried treatment after treatment. With every doctor's appointment and medical intervention, we desperately hoped to finally experience a breakthrough. But it didn't happen.

As the months passed, Emma naturally worried about whether she would be in constant pain her entire life. Would she be able to go to college, have a career, start a family, or pursue her dreams? Could she find a way to be happy?

We tried to help her cope with her hardship, including arranging for her to see psychologists, but the best remedy came from Emma herself. Emma chose to redesign her life and focus on what she *could do* to move forward with what she loved while managing her debilitating condition. One of her strategies was to immerse herself in school clubs (homeschooled children were allowed to join clubs), so she became active in speech and debate, mock trial, Model UN, and Future Farmers of America (FFA).

With FFA, Emma served as president of her school club, soon followed by being elected district president and county president. She showed dairy and beef cows, pigs, and goats at fairs. She won a state competition in vet science. She even persuaded us to buy her a cow. And we lived in suburbia! She had arranged for her cow to live at a local school in a fenced-in field that was a part of their agriculture program. It was therapeutic for Emma to get out in nature and be the caregiver for her cow every morning and evening.

Toward the end of Emma's junior year, after a year and a half of unrelenting pain, seeing over a dozen specialists, taking every imaginable diagnostic test, and trying more than thirty medical treatments, the sun finally appeared over the horizon, and she had a series of breakthroughs. First, a Botox regimen began to control her migraines. Then, Emma's doctor, the compassionate Dr. Hart, found a muscle relaxant—Flexeril (cyclobenzaprine)—that reduced the pain of her chronic daily headaches to a two- to four-level. This was still terrible but represented an improvement.

The last breakthrough was the diagnosis of the root cause of her condition. Dr. Hart concluded that Emma had hypermobile Ehlers-Danlos syndrome (hEDS), a genetic connective tissue disorder that weakens tendons and ligaments, among many other symptoms. It can cause a wide array of lifelong medical issues, including shoulder dislocations, migraines, and chronic daily headaches, as was the case with Emma. Though there wasn't a cure for hEDS, and we didn't know if her symptoms would degenerate over time, we at least had a name for her condition. We could now research case studies and join the worldwide EDS community to stay on top of medical advances.

Emma's progress had another significant benefit: She planned to return to in-person classes for her senior year. That lifted all of our spirits!

Emma enjoyed her senior year. She split her time between in-person and online classes. She was still coping with her chronic daily headaches every second she was awake, but at least she was establishing a semblance of normalcy: attending school, participating in clubs, hanging out with friends, and dreaming about college.

Toward the end of her senior year, Dr. Hart had Emma try an extended-release version of Flexeril that she could take once a day. He wanted to see if it would smooth out the uneven results of her three-times-a-day regimen. After Emma took her first dose, she wouldn't tell us how she felt. Her silence about her condition continued for three long days. Kristen and I were cautiously optimistic that maybe, just maybe, she was silent because the Flexeril had positive results, and she wanted to ensure it wasn't a fluke. We desperately hoped that was the case. Every step forward in her condition was priceless.

Emma finally revealed to us that her headache had gone down to a zero- to one-level. IT WAS PRACTICALLY NONEXISTENT!!! She had experienced a pain-free day for the first time in two and a half years! We didn't know if her improvement would last, but now she had proof that it was within the realm of possibility to control her condition. It was like the universe put its hand on her shoulder and told her: "We will get through this."

Remember when I wrote a few pages back that Emma was usually five chess moves ahead of me? Here's a prime example: During the latter part of her senior year, Kristen and I had to deal with the most challenging parental decision we ever had to make. Emma's journey over the last two and a half years—which made her feel like she was climbing a steep, jagged mountain covered in tacky glue—had led her to an audacious ambition: She wanted to spend her entire summer before college living out of her car as she drove across the country bingeing on national parks.

Emma revealed her full vision to us in a beautifully laid-out, eighty-slide PowerPoint presentation that could best be described as a detailed legal brief adorned with pictures of breathtaking mountains. She planned to start in Florida, drive up the East Coast, and head to California. On her journey back to Florida, she would travel through the South. For each day of her trip, she had a detailed itinerary of what she wanted to experience, which included a lot of hiking. She also created a budget that factored in food, gas, permits, and supplies, which she planned to self-fund. Her well-reasoned arguments for taking the trip *with our blessing* would have made Cicero proud.

What a seemingly impossible decision Kristen and I had to make. What if we said "yes" and something terrible happened? What if we said "no" and, besides Emma resenting us, she missed out on a coming-of-age opportunity that could have shaped the rest of her life? My inclination was to say "no." There was too much risk for my risk-averse brain to wrap its lobes around.

As we considered what to do, our hearts kept returning to Emma's life journey. Her whole life had prepared her for this moment. She was responsible, independent, and a problem-solver. After being held back for two and a half years by a wicked force out of her control, she felt compelled to explore the world. She needed to live for today because she didn't know what tomorrow would bring. She needed to find herself. Her arguments tugged at my spirit. I understood the place she was coming from.

Kristen and I soon accepted that we had to find a way to "yes." Emma's desire to take this trip wasn't a fleeting flight of fancy; this was coming from deep within her.

So we thought of every possible risk of taking the trip, and worked out plans to mitigate them as best we could. We examined her itinerary and negotiated adjustments. We planned to have Kristen join Emma on the first leg of her trip (a week traveling up the East Coast) to ensure she was fully prepared for her adventure. After that, Emma would connect with her sister, Audrey, for a few days in Colorado. I would then join Emma in Montana and travel with her to the West Coast. We even went to the extreme of draining some of our savings to buy Emma a new car equipped with all the latest safety features. We had to get to "yes" for our daughter and position her for success.

Emma went on her cross-country trip, living out of her car, and it transformed her life. She hiked some of the most gorgeous mountains in America. She experienced Death Valley, the Grand Canyon, the Atlantic and Pacific Oceans, the redwoods in California, and Yellowstone. During her trip, I took the following picture of Emma jumping off a cliff into the frigid, fiftyish-degree, crystal-blue water at stunning Crater Lake, Oregon. If a picture was ever worth a thousand words, this could be the one:

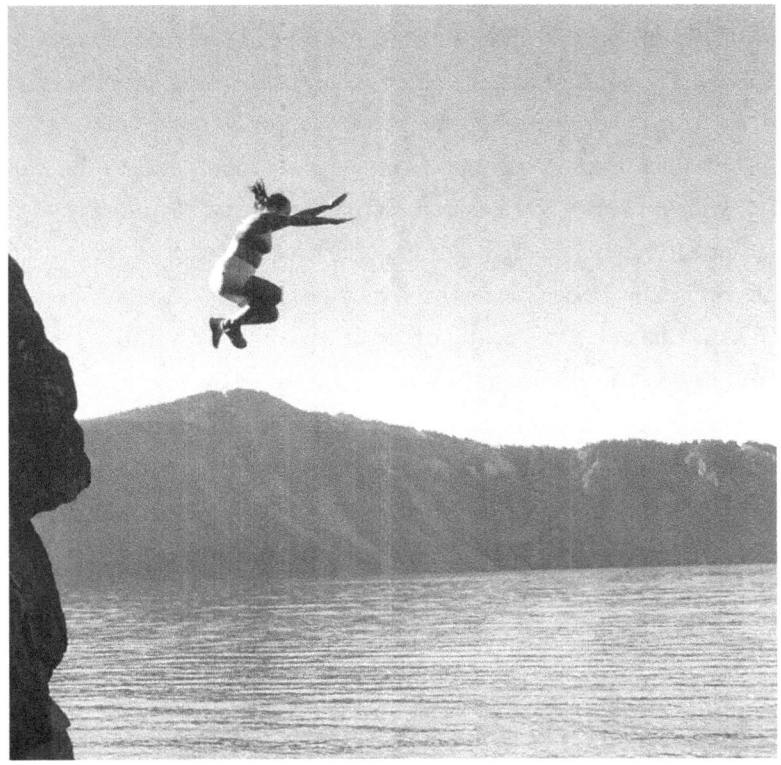

In my opening dedications, I mentioned that my children have taught me more about living than a thousand books could ever teach. That speaks to the wonderful gifts parenting two children can provide to a father. In the case of Emma, indulge me as I give you a glimpse into how she has inspired me.

I witnessed firsthand one of the most courageous examples of a will to live I've ever encountered. Seeing my daughter struggle daily with headaches for years but still maintain her zest for life was awe-inspiring. I think about her getting a perfect 800 on the verbal portion of her SAT exam while having a splitting headache. Or self-publishing a poetry book and writing and giving dozens of speeches in debate competitions, all while she was in excruciating pain. Somehow, she maintained a healthy detachment from the hell she was living through to tap into every ounce of resolve she had to mindfully engage with life as it was, not how she wished it to be.

I learned about the value of *experiencing* life. Emma's first road trip lit an adventurous fire within her that burns brilliantly to this day. As I write this, Emma is a junior in college. Her headaches are still under control (*knock, knock, knock*). She has completed three cross-country road trips, hiked alone in Alaska's Denali National Park for a week, and walked a four-hundred-mile solo backpacking trek along the Oregon coast. She's a certified SCUBA divemaster. And on and on. Sharing all her adventures could take up another book, and I hope she writes that book someday.

Perhaps most importantly, Emma seared within me one of life's most empowering truths. While she was sitting near the edge of a mountain cliff overlooking a valley during her first cross-country road trip, she had an epiphany: She realized that she controls her happiness. No other person or force, not even a vicious illness, has that control over her. Her joy is within her. That deep spiritual insight liberated her from the challenges in her life and positioned her to navigate the good and the stupid that will surely cross her path in the future.

I look at how she courageously chose her life-affirming, love-centered responses to her extreme obstacles and think, *My daughter figured out how to nurture the wonderful gift of her existence before graduating from high school, and I'm writing a book in my fifties to try to attain the same wisdom!*

When I reflect upon how Emma has lived her life, I can't think of a more perfect inspiration for what it means to have a Wellness Ethic mindset.

o  o  o

# CHAPTER 10

# Calm Psyche, Happy Lifey

Today, at this very moment, I am happy.

I got off to a great start this morning. I had a good night's sleep. I took a peaceful four-mile walk, followed by thirty minutes of cardio and a refreshing shower. I ate an oatmeal breakfast with fruit, walnuts, flaxseed, and soy milk. I fed Christopher McFluffer (our adopted stray cat). I then checked the mailing status of a relic-condition, thousand-year-old pair of Viking shears that I bought from an antiquities dealer. I'll admit it's an odd purchase, but I have a perfect spot for it reserved on a bookshelf in my office. I can't wait.

That launch to my day has flowed into what I'm doing now: living my life purpose by writing this chapter. To lift my spirits while I create, I'm savoring a heavenly cup of cinnamon spice tea and listening to the pleasing Tin Pan Alley sounds of Leon Redbone. There's just something about his music that brings me joy. It also inspires me to sing along, though I restrict my off-key singing performances to the privacy of my office due to a cease-and-desist order my family filed against me.

Right now, I have a perfect blend of purpose, challenge, and serenity. There could be many distractions. The bearish stock market is scrambling my retirement nest egg. American politics are maddening. Inaction on gun violence is horrible. But I focus on what I can control and detach my mind from the stupidity around me. By taking this approach, I'm not letting negativity occupy my consciousness. I'm doing that because, right now, it's time to be inspired. It's time to have fun toying with words. It's time to sing along with Leon Redbone. It's time to be happy.

## A Time to Be Happy

Happiness is an emotional state in which you feel positive and satisfied in the moment. Your mood is upbeat and agreeable. You feel good. Being happy is the desired outcome of having a Wellness Ethic mindset. But before we dive into this intriguing notion of having a "Wellness Ethic mindset," I'll set the stage by grounding us in four happiness fundamentals:

*Happiness can be experienced anywhere, anytime, and in any circumstance.* You could be happy doing things that just about any reasonable person would enjoy, such as relaxing on a recliner and losing yourself in a good book like *The Wellness Ethic*, or going to the beach to soak up the sun as the cool ocean breeze lulls you into a state of peaceful bliss, while you lose yourself in a good book like *The Wellness Ethic*. You could be happy doing the mundane, like cleaning a house. Just listen to music. That's probably all it'll take. You could also be happy at a wake as you celebrate a loved one's magnificent life with friends and family as tears and laughter flow.

*You have significant control over your happiness but not complete control.* Studies have shown that your genetics, life circumstances (age, health, relationships, life events, where you live, economic status), and intentional activity (what you do and your mindset) determine your happiness level. The percentage breakdown of how each factor impacts happiness varies across studies—one study showed that, on average, 50% of happiness is driven by genetics, 10% by life circumstances, and 40% by intentional activity.[1] But regardless of the exact percentages, the key takeaway is that you can influence a significant portion of your happiness by how you think and behave, what you pursue, and how you respond to life. That's empowering.

*Happiness is closely linked to fulfillment.* Your fulfillment—your deep satisfaction and inner peace—soars when you embrace your life purpose, love the universe of existence, and surrender to the ways of the universe. But those spiritual values also have a positive impact on happiness. When you volunteer and serve others, you feel happy that you contributed meaningfully to someone's life. When you celebrate a holiday with your family and feel love toward them, that feeling is often accompanied by joy.

*Happiness is linked to your physical wellness, and vice versa.* Do you feel good after a workout? Are you happier after a good night's sleep? From your own experience, you have probably felt the connection between physical wellness and happiness. Science also supports the relationship. A cross-sectional study showed that psychological well-being increases when people adopt healthy lifestyles, including being physically active, not smoking, and eating a healthy diet.[2]

The reverse also holds true: Happy people live healthier lives. Research has demonstrated that positive emotions can lead to better lifestyle choices and reduced stress, which can lower blood pressure, reduce the risk of stroke and heart disease, strengthen immunity, and improve longevity.[3]

## Happiness and the Wellness Ethic Mindset

A mind devoted to happiness—or Wellness Ethic mindset for our purposes—takes your thoughts and experiences, which start as neutral, and molds them to create the conditions for happiness. Something like this:

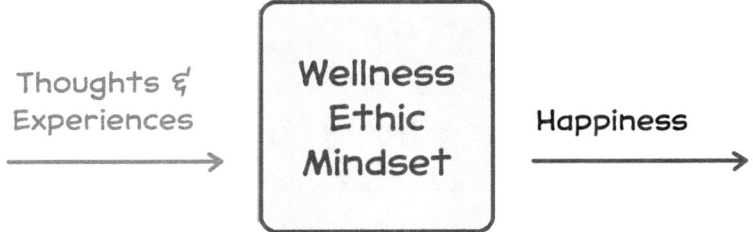

The process begins when thoughts and experiences enter your mind. Initially, they're neutral as they wait for your interpretation, influencing whether you feel happy, unhappy, or somewhere in the middle. Your SAGe wants your interpretation to generate as much happiness as possible. That's where the Wellness Ethic mindset comes into play.

A Wellness Ethic mindset, from an 80/20 perspective, consists of four elements. The first three—*positivity, mindful engagement,* and *healthy detachment*—are filters that thoughts and experiences travel through to help you shape what has entered your mind into a perspective that positions you for happiness. The positivity filter promotes an optimistic and enthusiastic approach to life. Mindful engagement is about experiencing the world with heightened awareness and appreciation. When you practice healthy detachment, you accept that the universe has positive and negative forces. You then choose to focus on what you can control—your thoughts and actions—while managing your emotions with what you can't. This helps maintain tranquility.

The fourth element of the Wellness Ethic mindset is *emotional intelligence* (EI). EI is the ability to manage your emotions and relate to the feelings of others. It serves as your mind's happiness regulator and is a catalyst for maintaining healthy emotions in an unpredictable world (where stupid things can happen). EI—a power tool of your SAGe—also suppresses your Mischief Mind, leading to better outcomes.

Here's an expanded version of the model to show how it comes together:

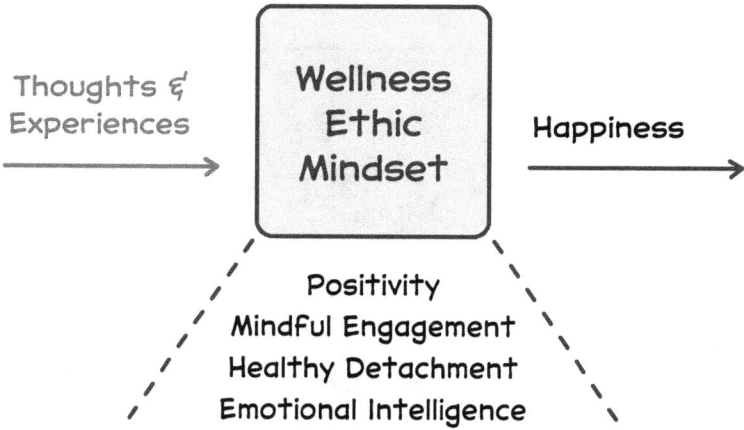

We'll now walk through the model. As we do so, think about how you can apply these mind-expanding concepts to bring more happiness into your life.

# Positivity
## *Illuminate the Moment*

Let's think about positive thinking. We'll start with the *enthusiastic* entrepreneur who takes a leap of faith and *courageously* launches a business because they *believe* in themselves and their vision. How about the *motivated* sports team that defeats Goliath because they *confidently* refuse to accept the limiting beliefs of their doubters? I still get goosebumps when I see highlights from the *inspired* 1980 US Olympic hockey team's improbable march to the gold medal, especially the final minutes of their *fearless* victory over the USSR hockey juggernaut. Positive thinking gives you *optimism* and *determination* to overcome obstacles and perform at your best. It *empowers* you.

Positive thinking also has a direct impact on your happiness. Happiness comes from positive emotions and states of mind like love, optimism, confidence, and inspiration, not hate, anger, doubt, or fear. Happiness is positive. Thinking that happiness could come from negativity would be as foolish as reading a medical claim denial letter and expecting to understand it without utilizing sleuthing skills that would put a World War II codebreaker to shame.

Since we're on the topic of insurance claims, isn't it irritating when you navigate an insurance carrier's customer avoidance phone system? You try every imaginable combination of menu options and phrases to coax the system to transfer you to a person. If you eventually succeed, you then get passed around from department to department. When I think about the battles I waged to get my daughter Emma's medical claims covered, I get so angry—

Stop! I must pull the emergency brakes on this happiness-derailing train of thought! As you painfully witnessed, negativity can seize your mind without warning. But with a simple redirect—like I did—you can make it vanish.

**You have a choice: Do you want to be a positive or negative person?** To boost your positivity (wise choice), I'll focus on three approaches: *develop a growth mindset, reframe automatic negative thought patterns*, and *make positivity your MO*. These approaches expand upon the techniques to nurture a positive mindset covered in chapter 6.

## Develop a Growth Mindset

Underpinning a SAGe's positive mindset is a devotion to growth. In her book *Mindset: The New Psychology of Success*, Carol Dweck introduced the concept of a growth mindset.[4]

A person with a growth mindset steps out of their comfort zone, leans into challenges, and takes calculated risks. They have a zest for self-improvement and seize opportunities that push their boundaries. By doing so, they unlock their vast potential. When setbacks occur, they are resilient and view failure as motivation to learn and grow rather than a reflection of their competence.

The opposite of a growth mindset is a fixed mindset. A person with a fixed mindset tends to be set in their ways, doesn't welcome constructive feedback, and is overwhelmed by difficulties. When they struggle, they get consumed by negativity and resist pivoting in new directions. As a result, they limit their growth and success, undermine their happiness, and deflate team morale.

To nurture a growth mindset, motivate yourself to get out of your comfort zone and embrace challenges (you'll figure things out along the way). Seek opportunities to learn (you can learn anything). Act upon feedback (it truly is a gift). Give yourself grace when you struggle, knowing that obstacles are a part of the growth process (everyone has struggled). If you do stuff like that, a growth mindset will become your default position. You'll approach opportunity (and life) with enthusiasm, and happiness often comes along for the ride.

A side note: The previous paragraph highlights why I placed the "Respond Perfectly to the Imperfect" and "Jack of No Change, Master of None" chapters at the beginning of *The Wellness Ethic*. They cover approaches that can help you implement learnings from this book. In the case of developing your growth mindset, you could use the Accept-Frame-Respond model in the moment to choose a growth-oriented frame and response to an opportunity. Or you could use change adoption techniques—affirmations, visual management, align support—to help make strengthening your growth mindset a daily priority. Revisit those chapters to see how they can help you grow.

## Reframe Automatic Negative Thought Patterns

Based on past experiences, you may feel negative about something without much thought. This can be helpful in dicey situations where every second counts. For example, if you were a caveman moseying about with another caveman and a saber-toothed tiger jumped out from the brush, you wouldn't want to complete a 5 Whys exercise to better understand the tiger's intentions. There's no time! Your life is at risk! You must quickly trip the other caveman, offer your sincere apology to said caveman, and then flee for your life!

But you want to be careful not to assign negativity to situations that don't need to be negative. This tendency, called *automatic negative thought patterns (ANTs)*, can lead to unhappiness and poor decisions. Some common ANTs are:

○ *All-or-Nothing Thinking:* You see a situation in black-and-white terms with no middle ground. Example: If you make a mistake, you view yourself as a complete failure who can't do anything right.

○ *Magnification and Minimization:* You blow things out of proportion. Examples: You think a setback is the world's end (magnification), or your achievement doesn't matter (minimization).

○ *Overgeneralization:* You draw broad conclusions from a single event. Example: You feel like you are not smart after failing a test.

○ *Jumping to Conclusions:* You immediately think the worst about a situation without objectively considering the facts. Examples: You think a hiring manager will reject you (mind reading), or you expect that a future event will turn out negatively (fortune-telling).[5]

To counter automatic negative thought patterns, focus on developing the habit of catching yourself in the moment when you're feeling negative. Then, objectively look at the truth of your situation and choose a positive, reality-based frame. Here are examples of ANTs with positive reframes:

| Negative Thought | Positive Reframing |
|---|---|
| I didn't execute perfectly. I'm a failure. (all-or-nothing thinking) | *I won't let perfect be the enemy of good. In fact, nothing is ever perfect. I will focus on what's right and build off of that. I am competent.* |
| Artificial intelligence will take my job. I won't be able to support my family. (fortune-telling) | *I'll focus on what I control: being proactive with my career and developing skills. The future has unlimited potential. I will find my path.* |
| My boss was critical of my work. She doesn't respect my abilities. (mind reading) | *Everyone has opportunities for improvement. I'll ask for her perspective on my strengths and development needs. I am very talented.* |

Negativity undermines happiness. If you're unsure about that, think of a time when you were happy *and* consumed with negativity. I am positive you won't be able to. Such an example would defy the way the mind works.

## Make Positivity Your MO

Illuminating each moment of your day with positivity will improve your life. Making positivity your modus operandi (MO)—how you operate—is well within your grasp. Here are three ways you can make positive thinking a habit:

*Use visual management and affirmations to remind yourself to be positive.* Place a note with the word "positivity" on your computer, bathroom mirror, or refrigerator. Create an affirmation and repeat it often, such as: "I am a positive thinker who sees my world through an optimistic lens." Be positive about being a positive person.

*Surround yourself with positivity; limit exposure to negativity.* Spend time with positive people; limit time with those who are not. Read inspiring books. Watch uplifting movies. Go on a news fast.

*Ask for support.* A friend or a family member can keep you honest by pointing out when you're being negative. A life coach or a therapist can help you maintain a positive outlook as you work through challenges.

The more you focus on positivity, the more positive your life will be.

# Mindful Engagement
## *Become One with the Moment*

Come take a stroll with me. But first, let's pause momentarily in my office, clear our minds, and just listen. We hear the breathtaking sound of the Modern Jazz Quartet's "I'll Remember April" pulsating from my Bose speakers, the perfect, uplifting blend of piano, vibraphone, bass, and drums.

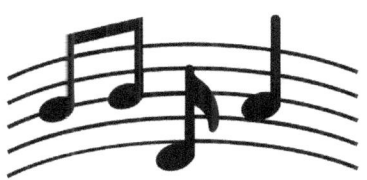

If you listen closely, you can isolate the sound of each instrument and appreciate its elegant contribution to the composition's soundscape. Take a deep, relaxing breath. Slowly exhale. Life is good.

We'll now walk toward my office door. Take a minute to notice the Benedict Arnold signed document from 1787 framed on the wall to the left.

It relates to Arnold's lawsuit against a former Loyalist comrade-in-arms. See the wrinkles and folds in the old document? I wonder how many hands this piece of paper passed through over the centuries, each person with a story to tell. Isn't it surreal that the infamous American Revolutionary War traitor signed this document as he tried to recover a debt originating from one of his many suspect business dealings? What a villainous character. I love history.

Let's step outside my office and head downstairs. We must stop to appreciate the exquisite painting in my stairwell: Sherrie Wolf's *Still Life with Claude Lorrain Landscape*.

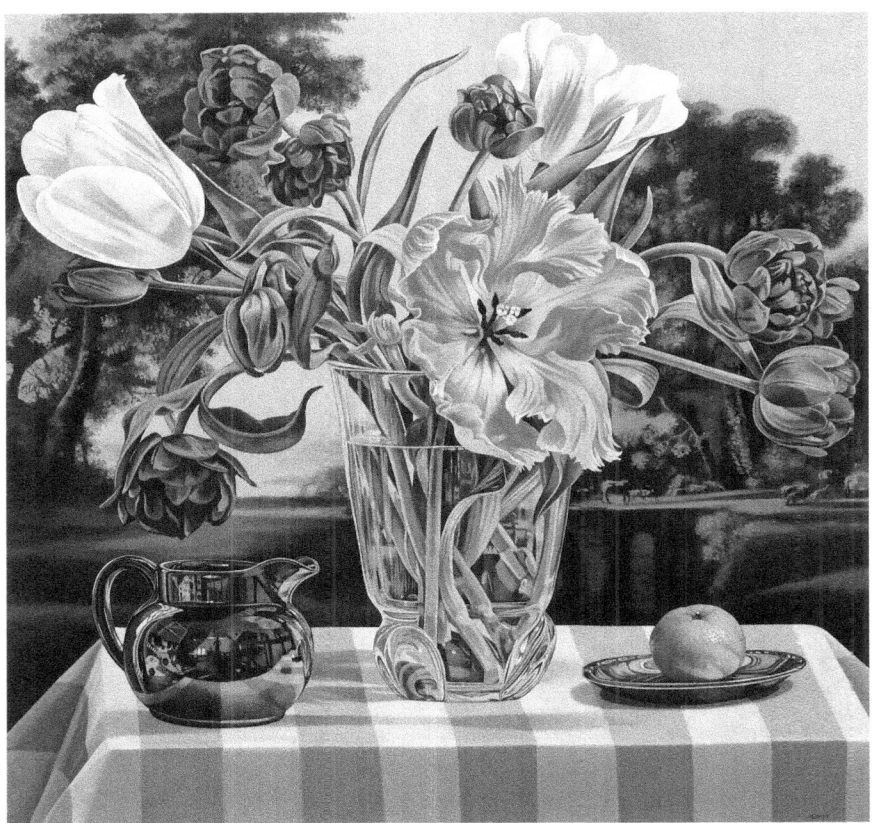

Sherrie is a photorealist painter who uses classic art as a backdrop to her still lifes. What a stunningly beautiful composition. I mean, look closely at the reflections and shadows dancing about the canvas. The detail and beauty of the flowers. The impeccable folds of the tablecloth. The crystal vase that looks like it was freshly filled with water moments ago. Notice how everything harmonizes perfectly, inviting you into Sherrie's wondrous imagination. I'm amazed that someone can create such splendor from a blank canvas. What a gift she has. I love getting lost in art.

Ready to move on? Probably not—there's still much more to discover in Sherrie's painting—but follow me as we head downstairs and walk to my back porch. I have something else I'd like you to experience.

All right, we're here. Simply relax as you look all around my backyard. Soak in the sounds and beauty of nature. Merge with the experience.

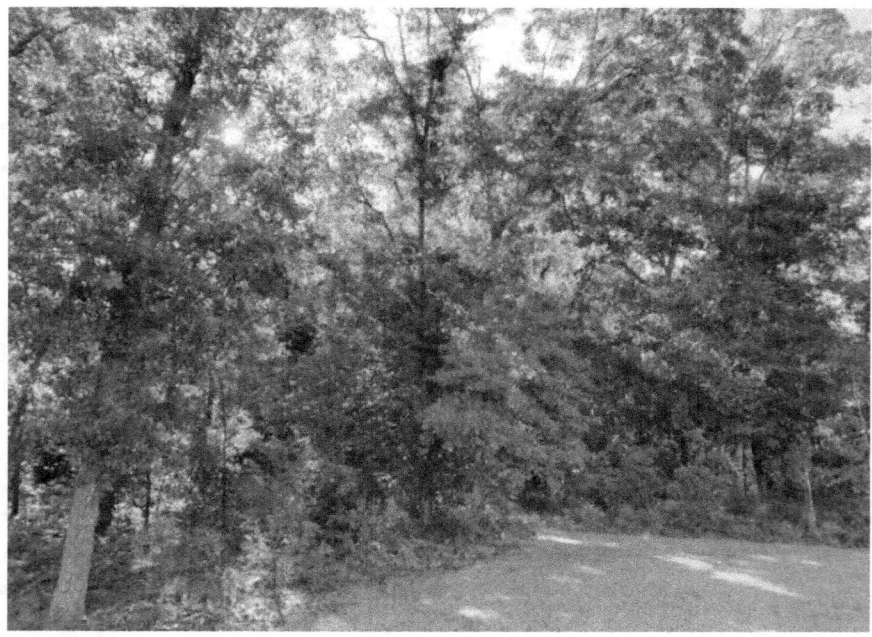

Nothing seems remarkable until you engage your senses. Did you hear the crow squawking? She must have seen something that delighted her. Look to the right and you'll see a row of oak trees that I planted. They were seedlings from the legendary Angel Oak tree on Johns Island, South Carolina. I love seeing them thrive in their new habitat.

Off to the left, there's a squirrel climbing a pine tree. I'm sure he has a purpose for what he's doing, or maybe not. Perhaps climbing the tree and being a squirrel is his purpose? Hmm. There's probably a profound lesson about the universe in that thought. We can think about it later.

Now close your eyes for five minutes. Listen to the sounds of nature and feel the warm breeze against your skin on this summer morning.

Okay, you can open your eyes now. I don't know about you, but I'm glad I took that mindful engagement tour. I found myself fascinated with the ordinary and the extraordinary. In fact, I would suggest it was all extraordinary. Even the simplest things, like seeing a tree's branches sway in the wind, were mesmerizing when I cleared my mind and became one with the moment. I found myself at peace. I wasn't judging anything. I wasn't even aware if I was happy or not. That wasn't the point. I just wanted to *be*. And after the experience, I feel less stress. I feel like I know what matters in my life. I feel happy.

Mindful engagement has many facets. To keep it simple, I'll focus on two types: *everyday mindfulness* and *flow (optimal experience)*.

## Everyday Mindfulness

Mindfulness is your SAGe's natural state of mind. When you are mindful, you immerse yourself in an experience, appreciating its nuances and connecting with its essence. You elevate your senses and tune out everything but the purity of your oneness with the experience before you. It's about love, nonjudgment, and accepting the experience for what it is—perfection in the moment.

Mindfulness is associated with the "love the universe of existence" spiritual value. When you're spiritual, you feel a sense of awe for the universe and the interconnectedness of all living things. A great way to do that is to mindfully engage with your experiences. Observe details. Focus on the wonder.

Give it a shot. Try mindfully engaging with a banana. Notice the shape and color. Feel the texture. Then, connect with the sensation of peeling it and the aroma and flavor as you eat it. When you swallow, dare to think about digestion and nutrients entering your body. Isn't that mind-blowing? And that's just a banana! The universe is miraculous, which is why we mindfully engage in its offerings.

If you practice mindfulness regularly, here's what will happen: You will reduce stress and feel calmer. You'll think more clearly. You will slow down the earth's spin and develop a healthier perspective on life. You'll feel gratitude for your blessings, some of which you may have taken for granted. You will be happier and more fulfilled. Mindfulness is that powerful.

There are many different approaches to practicing mindfulness. Perform an internet search, and you'll find an endless stream of free content, including videos, blog articles, and websites. You could also take a mindfulness class, utilize an app, or work with a mindfulness coach. As a resource for this book, I'll offer a six-step mindfulness approach:

○ *Step 1: Set your intention.* Determine your mindfulness objective and approach. Do you want to sit comfortably and engage in a guided meditation (instructor-led or pre-recorded) to bring calm to your life? Or do you want to guide yourself? Perhaps you'd enjoy a walk in nature, or maybe you want to savor the gift of every morsel during a meal?

○ *Step 2: Prime your environment for optimal focus.* Mute the devices. Get comfortable. Control anything—to the best of your ability—that could distract your senses from your mindfulness intention.

○ *Step 3: Position your mind for a fully immersive experience.* Take slow, deep breaths through your nose, at least three seconds for each inhale (use your diaphragm) and three seconds for each exhale. Clear your mind of all thoughts and sensations besides the feeling of air entering and leaving your body. If a thought enters your mind, gently push aside the distraction. Once your mind is calm, go to the next step.

○ *Step 4: Observe and engage.* Continue to breathe slowly and deeply at a comfortable level as you activate your senses and fuse with your experience. Notice the detail. Be sure not to judge what you're focused on. Step outside your mortal thoughts and operate at the level of purity. Be in awe. Be grateful. Be one. Just be.

○ *Step 5: Push aside interference.* Other thoughts outside your intention may enter your mind. That's not failure—an active mind is not used to operating at the level of mindful focus. When interference happens, acknowledge the intrusion, push it aside, and refocus. If you don't return to a mindfulness state, go back to Step 3 and focus your attention on your breathing. Then, when you're ready, resume Step 4.

○ *Step 6: Return and reflect.* Once your experience is over, reflect on it. Did you learn anything? Does the world seem grander and your problems smaller? Do you feel happy and at peace? Soak in the positive energy and allow it to carry you forward throughout your day.

A mindfulness experience can last a few minutes or longer. It's your choice. As you practice mindfulness, you'll train your brain to become more attentive to your surroundings. You'll notice and appreciate the fullness of your experiences, even the little things you might have overlooked in the past. You'll find wonder everywhere, often without trying.

Start today. Mindfully engage for at least five minutes and see what it does for you. Moving forward, do you want to schedule a daily mindfulness break on your calendar? Or set a recurring alarm on your phone to help you build a mindfulness habit?

## Flow (Optimal Experience)

I was playing shortstop on my junior varsity baseball team. It was an ordinary game, but then something remarkable happened that I still remember vividly forty years later. A ball was hit way over my head into the outfield. When you've played sports long enough, you can tell immediately whether you have a shot at making a play. I knew my odds of catching the ball were between zero and zilch. Hopefully, the outfielder would record the out.

But without thinking, I found myself sprinting in the direction where I thought the ball was headed. I didn't look up to track it because something inside me knew if I looked up, I would lose precious milliseconds of momentum, eliminating any chance of snagging the ball. So I ran as fast as I could.

Still, the urge to look up wouldn't go away—I had to know if I was tracking the ball! *No! Don't look up, you fool! Keep running! Keep running!* Again, intuition stopped me—I couldn't lose a millisecond! So I continued my mad dash for what seemed like eternity, sprinting and sprinting, not sure if I was tracking the ball, waiting for just the perfect moment to—

*LOOK UP!* I quickly glanced over my shoulder and saw the blur of the ball whiz over my head on a collision course with the ground. I was too late to make the catch. Argh! I wasn't fast enough!

But something compelled me to dive for the ball anyway. I didn't plan to dive. I was absolutely sure the play was over. Yet I found myself airborne with my glove stretched out as far as I could reach. And I caught the ball!

As my bones crashed to the ground in a heap, with the ball protruding from my glove's webbing, I held firm. One millisecond slower, and I wouldn't have made what I've told my family was the greatest catch in sports history. They know not to laugh anymore when I repeat the claim, which happens at least semiannually, because they understand I'm quite serious. I was there. I caught that ball!

The play took about five seconds to complete. But for those five seconds, I was "in the zone" where time and space were suspended, my focus was flawless, and every ounce of talent I had was fully activated to meet the moment. Anything less—even one tiny miscalculation or stumble—and I wouldn't have made what is widely regarded as the greatest catch in sports history, for those who see it that way, which, sadly, is a population of one. Oh well. At least I'll always have memories of the most thrilling five seconds of my life!

Mihaly Csikszentmihalyi wrote an influential book about being "in the zone" called *Flow: The Psychology of Optimal Experience.* Csikszentmihalyi described flow as "the state in which people are so involved in an activity that nothing else seems to matter; the experience itself is so enjoyable that people will do it at great cost, for the sheer sake of doing it."[6] That may explain why people climb dangerous peaks, BASE jump, or engage in other risky activities.

But you don't need to risk your life to have an optimal experience where you lose your sense of self. I've experienced flow while writing this book, playing sports, and working on projects at my job. As you train yourself to become more mindful, you'll learn how to block out distractions and fully engage in the moments that make up your day. And sometimes you'll find yourself *in the zone* where you lose track of time as you seamlessly immerse in the task at hand. When that happens, your activity will seem natural and effortless, you'll perform at your peak, and you'll love every second of it.

Several elements go into creating the conditions for a "flow" experience. To simplify flow, I'll focus on four key ones, which are derived from Csikszentmihalyi's work:

○ *Engage in a rewarding task that has a goal.* The task should have a clear objective that intrinsically motivates you. It should also be something you enjoy. Example: playing a competitive sport.

○ *Strike the balance between skill and action.* The task should be challenging enough that you need to leverage your talents in a focused manner to be successful, but not so hard that the task is impossible. Example: completing a difficult work task.

○ *Have an immediate feedback loop.* You should know how you're doing throughout the task and whether you're trending toward success. Example: taking a timed test.

○ *Block out all distractions.* Your focus and engagement should be such that the rest of the world recedes to the background. Example: playing a musical instrument.

When you combine those elements, sometimes you'll experience flow, or maybe not—flow is unpredictable. But the more you practice mindfulness and set the conditions for an optimal experience (especially blocking out distractions), the more you'll engage with your experiences. That's a win, whether flow happens or not. But just so we're clear: If you play baseball and get into a flow state, you'll still never top my catch. So don't even try. Or if you do try and happen to succeed, don't tell my family. I'm good either way.

## Healthy Detachment
### *Be Tranquil in the Moment*

I haven't watched the news for two weeks. I had to commit to a news fast for my mental health—it was making me sad and angry. The news was like a radioactive meltdown, releasing its toxic effects long after the initial calamity. Climate change was especially toxic to my psyche. Drought. Floods. Hurricanes. Tornadoes. Death. Destruction. I don't need to go on—we're living it. And it will get worse. Then I think about the leaders who fail to take bold action or the denialism about humans being the primary cause of climate change—I'm getting a headache. I need to be stoic.

### Stoicism
Stoicism, which originated in Greece around 300 BCE, is an ancient philosophy that espouses wisdom, courage, moderation, and justice as the pillars of a well-lived life. Among its many benefits, it can help you maintain inner peace and clarity of purpose during situations that could drag you down, which is what I'll focus on in this section.

Stoicism encourages you to use an enlightened perspective to accept and manage your emotions so they serve you. By doing so, you avoid becoming overwhelmed by circumstances out of your control. It's like having a shield when arrows are flung your way.

Today, Stoicism has experienced a revival as influential leaders have embraced its ethos to thrive in an unpredictable world (where stupid things can happen). The Wellness Ethic will focus on three Stoic-inspired perspectives that help you detach from a situation's negative energy by fostering a healthy attitude about how life works and what you can control. As a point of clarity, Stoicism doesn't advocate suppressing your emotions but instead promotes dealing with them productively so they serve your well-being.

## Stoicism: Detach from Negative Forces

One of the guiding principles of *The Wellness Ethic* is that you control your perspective regarding what is happening around you. You can choose to have a positive or negative outlook.

> *Begin in the morning by saying to yourself, I shall meet with the busybody, the ungrateful, arrogant, deceitful, envious, unsocial. All these things happen to them by reason of their ignorance of what is good and evil . . . I can neither be injured by any of them, for no one can fix on me what is ugly, nor can I be angry with my kinsman, nor hate him. For we are made for cooperation . . . To act against one another then is contrary to nature.*
>
> —Marcus Aurelius, Roman emperor, Stoic philosopher

The Stoic understands that they alone can't alter the course of the world, nor can they prevent the malcontent from trying to cast a loveless shadow over others through their insensitive words or misguided deeds.

The Stoic expects that they will encounter negative forces throughout their day, so they're not surprised when they do. When it occurs, they accept that things happen in life they can't control. They then detach themselves from the negative energy by focusing on what they can control: maintaining inner tranquility and acting within their sphere of influence. The Stoic knows that negative forces always seek to occupy their mind, but it's their choice whether they allow them in.

## Stoicism: Detach from Wants

A Stoic wants stuff just like everyone else. They don't necessarily desire a spartan existence. However, the wisdom in a Stoic's approach to "wants" is that they restrict their desires to what is within their control to attain, and they temper their wants, understanding that they already have everything they need.

> *Think not so much of what you lack as to what you have: but of the things you have, select the best, and then reflect how eagerly you would have sought them if you did not have them.*
> —Marcus Aurelius

The Stoic sees good all around them. They appreciate their blessings and don't take anything for granted. They avoid the fool's folly of desiring something excessive or out of reach. They know that's not the path to happiness; it's the path to disappointment and sometimes despair.

## Stoicism: Detach from Outcomes

A Stoic understands that they always have control over their response to a given situation but not necessarily the outcome of that response.

> *Some things are in our control and others not. Things in our control are opinion, pursuit, desire, aversion, and, in a word, whatever are our own actions. Things not in our control are body, property, reputation, command, and, in one word, whatever are not our actions.*
> —Epictetus, Greek Stoic philosopher

The Stoic chooses responses to life that align with their values and have the most potential to create a positive outcome. That is what they control. If the actual result is out of their control, they emotionally detach from it. That doesn't mean they don't care. They still do everything they can to achieve an objective, but they won't sacrifice their mental well-being for a result beyond their control. They emotionally invest in what they own, which is their mindset and their actions.

## Stoicism in Action

When I loop back to my climate change example that I shared earlier and apply a Stoic mindset, I believe the following:

> *I need to focus on what I control. I will be a good steward of the environment and urge others to do the same. I will be a change agent who looks for ways to play an active role in environmental causes (be engaged, not enraged). The global suffering caused by climate change is horrific, but it is out of my control. To be happy, I need to focus on my positive influence on the environment. That's within my control.*

That positive and realistic framing helps me keep a healthy perspective about an issue that could, otherwise, crush my spirit each day.

Think about situations where adopting a Stoic mindset would make you happier. Meditate on it. Then, embrace the mindset (try change adoption techniques we've covered previously to help with that intention—visual management, affirmations, others). If you slip into negativity, be self-aware, summon your SAGe, and frame a healthier mindset. That is always within your control.

# Emotional Intelligence
### *Regulate Happiness in the Moment*

Oh, the times at work when I desperately wanted to give someone a piece of my mind. Those were moments when I was wronged, and my emotions shot past the boiling point as quickly as a cup of water tossed into the sun. But thankfully, I rarely acted upon the urgings of my impulsive Mischief Mind. I was emotionally intelligent before I even knew that was a thing.

To this day, I regret the few times I lashed out—I accomplished nothing and looked quite foolish in the process of accomplishing nothing. Such was the case when I had an epic quitting moment at Little Caesars Pizza in high school. I worked there for two years. Then, one evening, several employees quit after a falling out with the owner, including my brother and his girlfriend, who was the manager of the joint. I had to defend their honor.

So I stormed into the owner's office and let him have it. My teenage brain came up with a bunch of idiotic reasons why I thought he ran a lousy pizza franchise. I was on a roll. It was brutal. I then handed in my apron and quit! How do you erase such an event from your mind? Think about it. My epic job-quitting moment occurred as a teenager and involved defiantly handing in an apron. An apron! A person doesn't recover from that.

Now, when I look back at the times when I was emotionally charged but kept the bigger picture in mind and exercised restraint, I never have regrets. A good example occurred early in my GE career when I was told I didn't get the highest rating in a performance review because the leader didn't know if I was "executive material." I had hit the ball out of the park on every goal that year, but he reserved the "outstanding" rating for those who met his arbitrary "executive" criteria. Apparently, I fell short. I always liked this leader, but wow. In his eyes, there was a ceiling on my potential. That was good to know.

Though I didn't internalize his misguided drivel, I was still upset he thought that way about me. That's when my emotional intelligence kicked in. I was pursuing other career opportunities and needed to remain in good standing at my current job for reference purposes, so I calmed my emotions and bit my furious tongue. Soon, I landed a position at another GE business. Two and a half years later, I left GE and joined Bank of America at the executive level. I'll admit that was gratifying (I am human, usually).

It was a good reminder to never underestimate someone's potential, especially your own.

## The Fundamentals of Emotional Intelligence

After I read Daniel Goleman's book *Emotional Intelligence*, I knew it was going to be a game changer for my relationships and overall happiness. Emotional intelligence (EI) is the ability to recognize and regulate one's emotions, as well as the ability to engage effectively with the feelings of others. To make EI accessible and actionable, I'll focus on four elements: self-awareness, self-management, social awareness, and relationship management, which are derived from Goleman's work.[7]

Emotional intelligence begins with *self-awareness* of positive and negative emotions. When you are emotionally intelligent, you're in touch with your feelings and understand how they affect your thoughts and behavior. You savor positive emotions like joy, compassion, hope, gratitude, love, and serenity. You're also aware of mood shifts and their triggers, recognizing that negative emotions such as anger, anxiety, jealousy, and frustration undermine your happiness and ability to relate to others.

Self-awareness then leads to *self-management* of your feelings to maintain emotional well-being. When you are in a positive emotional state, you are happier, of course, but you also improve your ability to foster healthy relationships, defuse difficult situations, and make better decisions.

If your emotional state isn't where it needs to be, what can you do to get it there? You could apply a Stoic mindset and detach from negative forces. Or summon your SAGe and work through the Accept-Frame-Respond steps or the 5 Whys to get underneath what's driving your emotions and how best to regulate them. You could also talk with a friend to help sort out how you feel, or calm your mind through deep breathing, meditation, and exercising.

Once you're in a productive emotional state, if you're relating with others, you can then focus on the next step: *social awareness*. What are the emotional states of the people you're dealing with? Are they positive? If not, what negative emotions are present, what's driving them, and how are they impacting your relationship? When you are socially aware, you empathize with others. You seek to understand their feelings, needs, and perspectives without passing judgment. You pay attention to verbal and nonverbal cues. You are also in tune with group dynamics and social norms and how they influence a person's emotions and behaviors.

After factoring in social awareness, you are then ready for *relationship management,* which is the process of relating with others to achieve a positive outcome. Considering the emotions of the involved parties is critical in this step. Someone who is emotionally hurt or angry probably won't relate effectively until those emotions are mitigated.

To bring emotional intelligence to the forefront of a conversation, use your words and demeanor to convey authentic empathy, care, and partnership. Here are examples of phrases you could use to foster a spirit of cooperation:

O *Please help me understand more about what you're experiencing.*

O *How do you feel about what happened?*

O *I can appreciate how you feel. If I were in the same situation, I would also be frustrated. I want to work together to make this better.*

O *That situation can be challenging. What do you think is the root cause of the issue?*

O *How can I support you during this difficult time? Is there anything I can do better?*

O *I always value your perspective, even if we don't agree on everything. But if we keep the lines of communication open, I'm confident we'll be able to work through this.*

O *I'm truly sorry if my words hurt you. That wasn't my intention.*

○ *I would love to work together and find a path forward that meets our needs. Do you have any thoughts on how we could do that?*

○ *Thank you for your honesty. I know it can be difficult to give constructive feedback. And please continue to give me feedback moving forward. I take it seriously.*

A person with high emotional intelligence genuinely cares about others. They communicate openly and respectfully. They manage their own emotions and promote productive emotions within others. They admit when they are at fault, build trust, and resolve conflicts. A person with high EI nurtures healthy relationships and finds pathways to win-win outcomes.

When the emotional charge in a relationship is positive, both parties are positioned to bring their best to their interactions. Better results are achieved, and the experience is more enjoyable. Emotional intelligence is a superpower.

**Happiness is not an external phenomenon. It is already within you. But if you struggle with happiness, consider professional support. Seeking help for something that challenges you is a sign of inner strength.**

○ ○ ○

## Move Forward on Your Wellness Ethic Journey!

(1) Complete the Wellness Ethic mindset assessment below to determine how well your mindset operates at the SAGe level to bring happiness into your life. Then, document your improvement focus (include change adoption techniques as appropriate).

Current State: *Rate how well you practice each Wellness Ethic mindset element. Use a scale of 1 to 10, with 1 = "quite lousy" and 10 = "extremely well." Circle the score(s) you want to focus on.*

| Wellness Ethic Mindset | Current State |
|---|---|
| Positivity | |
| Mindful Engagement | |
| Healthy Detachment | |
| Emotional Intelligence | |
| Improvement & Change Adoption Focus | |
| | |

(2) Advanced Topics (going beyond the 80/20): Do a deep dive into the "science of happiness" and "positive psychology" by searching the internet, listening to podcasts, or reading books. Becoming a student of happiness will serve you well (and it's a great way to flex your growth mindset).

# Mark's Example

(1) Complete the Wellness Ethic mindset assessment below to determine how well your mindset operates at the SAGe level to bring happiness into your life. Then, document your improvement focus (include change adoption techniques as appropriate).

| Wellness Ethic Mindset | Current State |
|---|---|
| Positivity | 8 |
| Mindful Engagement | (6) |
| Healthy Detachment | 7 |
| Emotional Intelligence | 8 |
| Improvement & Change Adoption Focus | |

With the fast pace of my life, I need to slow down and mindfully engage to ensure I'm getting the most out of each moment. To practice mindful engagement, I'll schedule a time at noon each day to take a break and engage for at least ten minutes. It may take the form of radically appreciating art, observing nature, or something else—there are an infinite number of ways to engage mindfully!

From a change adoption standpoint, the key will be to schedule a time in my calendar so I'm automatically prompted. This will help me establish the mindfulness habit.

# The Body

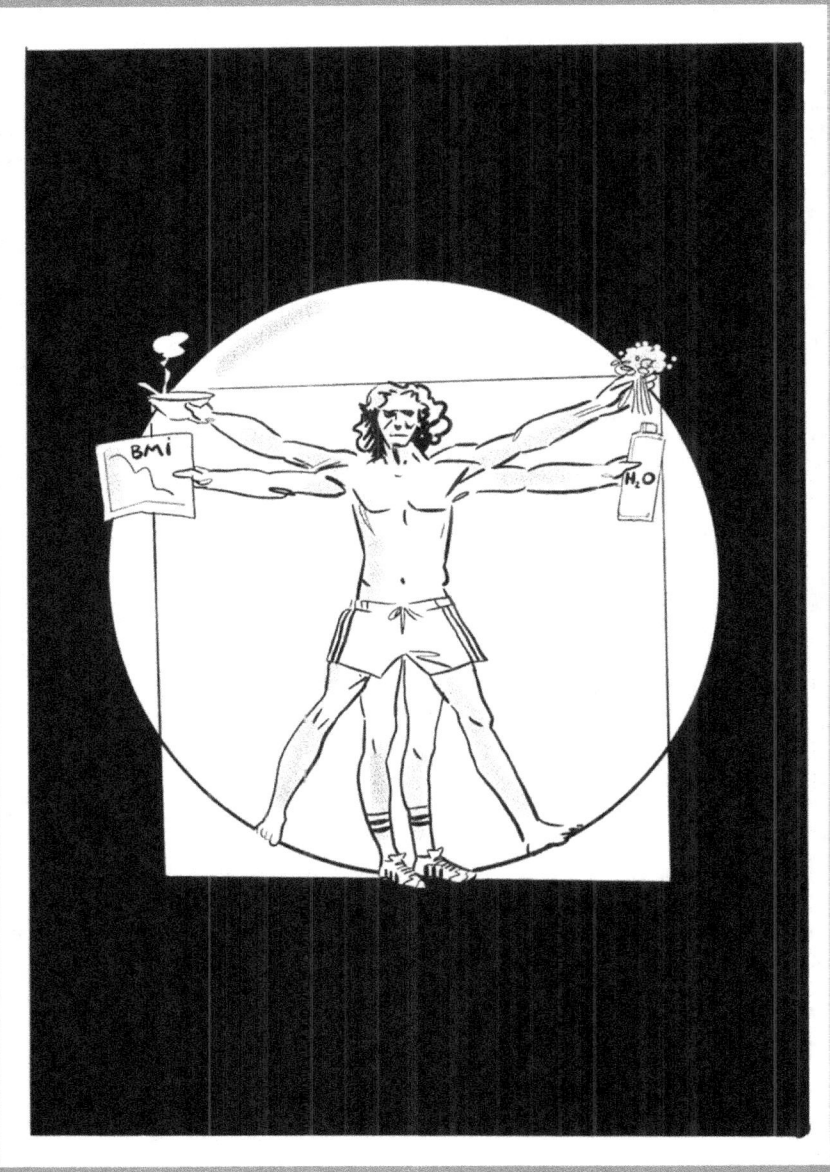

# CHAPTER 11

# A Story of Inspiration

I was taking a beeline to Burnoutville. It was the fall of 2022, and I was putting in the hours at my job, both weekdays and weekends. For decades, I had tried to block job-related slogging on weekends, but the corporate overwork virus always penetrated my firewall and exploited my vulnerabilities.

Throughout my career, I worked at companies with leaders who struggled to say "no" to lower priorities to free up capacity for the more important ones. When you're overcommitted, you spin rather than thrive. But, alas, spinning was my reality, and work would hemorrhage into the weekends.

So during my weekends, I would spend quality time with my family (nonnegotiable), and my side hustles would duke it out with my corporate obligations. I usually struck a decent balance, but not this time. My job dominated my life at the expense of writing *The Wellness Ethic*. Chapters that should have taken a month to complete were taking quadruple the time. I was miserable.

In a futile attempt to get back on track, I woke up on weekdays at 3:00 a.m. instead of my usual 4:00 a.m. to squeeze in more writing time. That turned out to be a stupid move. The sleep deprivation made me sluggish. Workouts were cut short. My diet became undisciplined. I gained weight. The quality of my writing nose-dived. Who would have thought an hour less of sleep could be so destructive? My life—as I had designed it—wasn't working. I needed to shake things up. It was time to go on a quest.

I love the concept of a quest. It's an engaging gamification technique that can be incredibly motivating. In a quest, you go on a mission to attain something meaningful. You encounter obstacles on the journey and must use your talents and resources to overcome them. Through those trials, you feel alive because you're challenged. You're growing. You're being rewarded. You're having fun. A good quest pushes your boundaries but stays within the realm of possibility.

For my quest, I decided to travel to Boston, Massachusetts, accompanied by my daughter Emma, and walk two marathons over a weekend (jogging them would have been too rough on my knees). The first marathon would take us 26.2 miles from Concord and Lexington to the Old North Church in downtown Boston to retrace, in reverse, the legendary patriot Paul Revere's midnight ride at the beginning of the American Revolutionary War ("The British are coming! The British are coming!"). The second would be a marathon walk around Walden Pond, a site made famous by Henry David Thoreau's nineteenth-century literary masterpiece *Walden*.

To help connect spiritually to the history of my surroundings, I down-loaded two audiobooks—Thoreau's *Walden* and *American Spring: Lexington, Concord, and the Road to Revolution* by Walter R. Borneman—and planned to listen to them during the walks.

This was shaping up to be an epic quest. By committing to it, I would need to train for two months to prepare my body, which would motivate me to become more disciplined with my diet and exercise routine. I needed that. And by being in the backyard of so much history and inspiration, I hoped to channel the wisdom to help me address my work-life balance issues to get my book back on track.

Our first marathon walk took place on a gorgeous Saturday morning in October. Autumn in New England is an experience to treasure. Clouds of silvery mist blanket the ponds and lakes as the sun rises. A kaleidoscope of colorful foliage adorns the trees. Cool, refreshing air invigorates your lungs. And on the weekends, people flock to the villages to revel in the last gasp of pleasant weather before winter barges in, creating a frigid, snow-covered habitat that only skiers and penguins can endure.

But Emma and I would let the natives worry about suffering through the long, dark winter and being unable to step outside their houses for five months without losing an extremity to frostbite. We were here to walk. A lot.

We started in Concord, walked through the town, and admired the beautiful colonial homes. We then entered Minute Man National Historical Park to walk the Battle Road Trail, which tracked the British Army's march to Lexington and Concord in 1775. We trekked across marshes and fields, encountering historical landmarks, including where the British captured Paul Revere, and watched reenactment soldiers fire muskets.

After the trail, we walked through Lexington. We stumbled across a Korean festival and enjoyed delicious bubble tea smoothies. We bought fresh apple cider doughnuts at a farmers' market a few miles later. Eating apple cider doughnuts on a fall day is a New England rite of passage. It reminded me of growing up in Upstate New York. I was glad Emma got to experience it.

We reached Boston's Old North Church in the evening, which completed our marathon. It was such an enjoyable experience.

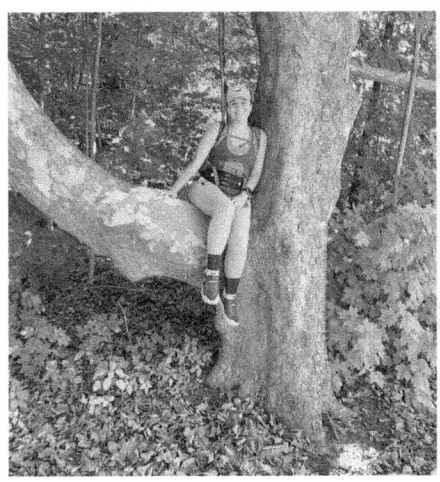
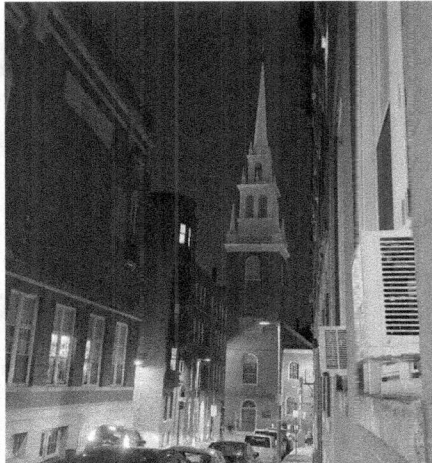

Emma befriends a tree—Concord, MA     Old North Church—Boston, MA

I had intended to listen to the *American Spring* audiobook for most of the walk, but that plan fell by the wayside. I was having too much fun exploring with Emma. Still, I was deeply moved during the few hours I listened to the book and soaked in the aura of sacrifice emanating from my surroundings.

I thought about how the revolutionaries risked their lives against improbable odds to free the American colonies from tyranny. They overcame setbacks for years as the revolution teetered on the edge of collapsing due to their inferior supply of troops, artillery, and funding. They were David against three Goliaths. But it didn't matter. They prevailed because they had something infinitely more valuable than resources—they had a noble purpose.

I then juxtaposed the struggles of the American revolutionaries against the struggles I was experiencing writing my book, and my challenges seemed small. I knew I could overcome them to realize my dream. I needed that healthy perspective at that very moment in my writing journey.

**Obstacles are to be expected—they are a part of living and doing—but a noble purpose provides the inspiration to carry on.**

The next day, Emma and I drove ten minutes from our hotel to Walden Pond to attempt our second walking marathon. I didn't know if my creaky, fiftyish body would make it, but I looked forward to the adventure. Walden Pond is breathtaking. See for yourself:

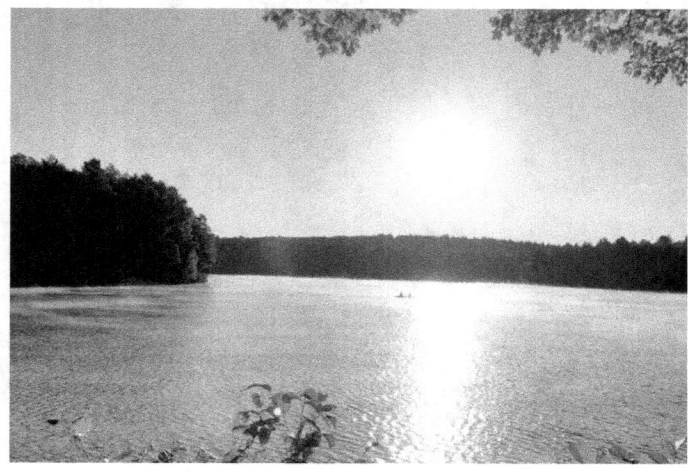

The pond's perimeter is approximately 1.7 miles, so round and round and round we went, and when we'd stop, well, it would be after 26.2 miles if my body held up! I imagine today's Walden Pond is close to how it appeared to Thoreau in the 1840s when he built his minimalist house near the pond's shore and began to write his timeless classic. For this walk, I logged three hours of the *Walden* audiobook between talking with Emma and pondering my place in the universe.

Walking in Thoreau's footsteps and listening to his teachings inspired me to merge my identity with the life around me as if we were a single organism. I watched industrious chipmunks forage for food to ready themselves for winter, just like their ancestors had done for millions of years. I passed by people from other lands and walks of life, traversing the Walden trails to find meaning. I looked into their eyes and understood that we shared a love for Mother Nature and humanity. That spiritual connection moved me. It tripled my conviction that we must respect our planet and coexist peacefully with others.

Emma and I finished the marathon. Two for two! The months of preparation paid dividends. As I completed the marathons, I expected to encounter physical obstacles, but my body held up wonderfully. For an old geezer like me, not bad. Not bad at all.

The quest served its purpose: My mind, body, and spirit were reenergized. The marathon training got my exercise and diet back on track. I bolstered my healthy perspective toward struggle and my commitment to advance confidently in the direction of my dreams. I even rethought my relationship with corporate America.

In the *Walden* audiobook, Thoreau provided profound wisdom that shifted my perspective on work-life balance. In his words, "The cost of a thing is the amount of what I call life, which is required to be exchanged for it, immediately or in the long run."

I decided that my dreams were too precious to be exchanged for long work hours. I had to exert more control over my time in corporate America, regardless of the priorities leaders assigned to me. I vowed to immunize against the corporate overwork virus by influencing my company's strategies, negotiating due dates, delegating more, and easing back on the extra work I imposed on myself in the spirit of "going above and beyond." (Postscript: My work pivots were successful. After the trip, my weekend work was reduced by around 90%.)

I needed an IV infusion of inspiration to help me blast out of the doldrums, and this trip provided that. I achieved many positive outcomes. But one outcome trumped them all: I created a shared memory with my daughter that we'll talk about for the rest of our lives. That got to the heart of the meaning of my life more than anything else. It was the true prize of completing my quest. I am so blessed.

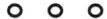

# CHAPTER 12

# Healthy Living Tastes Great and Is More Fulfilling

Let's chat about our bodies. I know what you're thinking. But don't worry. I'm not going there in our "chat about our bodies." Though it would be a wildly entertaining read to see how I stumbled through a description of how babies are made. For *The Wellness Ethic*, our 80/20 exploration of the body will center around the life satisfaction equation (Life Success = Feeling Love + Sharing Love = Wellness) and your physical health's role in helping to make the math work in your favor.

As a disclaimer, I won't provide prescriptive health advice in this chapter—I'll defer to your doctors. That's not a cop-out. It's recognizing that the human body is a ridiculously complex organism with approximately 37.2 trillion cells.[1] Offering customized advice that would optimize the performance of your cells is beyond my capabilities. Now, if your cell count were 31.45 trillion or less, that would be an entirely different ballgame.

Why does focusing on your body matter? If you want to thrive, optimizing your health to the best of your ability is required. Your health influences your vitality, the quality of your experiences, and your lifespan, which all impact your capacity to feel and share love. To bring stats into the picture, a 2018 Harvard study found that people who adopted healthy habits in adulthood—exercising, eating a healthy diet, not smoking, drinking moderately, and maintaining a healthy weight—"could prolong life expectancy at age 50 years by 14.0 and 12.2 years in female and male US adults compared with individuals without any of the low-risk lifestyle factors."[2]

Those results probably don't surprise you. But even if you make perfect health choices, the yellow brick road you follow during your wellness journey is never on a straight and even path. Expect potholes and bends, and witches and flying monkeys. Still, even when your health is challenged, living a long and happy life can be possible. Millions of people with debilitating conditions find meaningful ways to nurture the wonderful gift of their existence. They strive to live their healthiest life possible by focusing on what they can control.

Healthy living isn't always easy. I won't pretend otherwise. In my case, I must fight my competitive-eating-inspired temptation to strap on a bib and inhale an entire apple kuchen once it leaves the oven. I don't like visiting the doctor. I could come up with a list of five thousand things I'd rather do than lift weights, and that inventory would include cleaning the gunk out of a sink drain. Those physical wellness counterforces can find devious ways to score points against my wellness, even when my health-conscious SAGe is in the game. Imagine what it's like when my Mischief Mind is refereeing!

But your SAGe is mightier than your Mischief Mind when it's empowered with the know-how to steer you down a healthy path. That leads us to a captivating model—surprise, surprise! The Wellness Ethic's *STEER* model captures the heart of physical wellness: **S**cience, **T**reat, **E**at, **E**xercise, and **R**est.

## STEER Physical Wellness Model

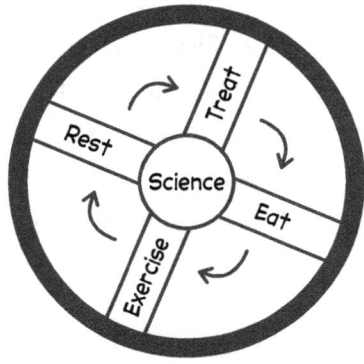

You will STEER your body in the healthiest direction—constrained by what you can control—if you trust but verify what the experts recommend and put that knowledge to use (*science*), practice preventive care and seek medical intervention when necessary (*treat*), align your diet to promote health (*eat*), regularly engage in physical activity (*exercise*), and allow your body adequate time to recharge (*rest*).

Healthy living may seem intimidating, especially if you have neglected your health. But you've been building confidence up to this point in your Wellness Ethic journey. You know the complicated can be broken down into nutritious, bite-sized nuggets. You understand that a two-mile walk begins with a single step. Remember when we covered how you're empowered to choose your SAGe-inspired response to life? And the change adoption practices we reviewed that enable lasting change? We'll bring all that stuff to bear to help you STEER your life in a healthy direction. You're ready for this. So strap on your OSHA-approved safety goggles and follow me to the science lab.

## Science – Treat – Eat – Exercise – Rest

Truth can be liberating. It can be a growth catalyst that moves your life forward. Truth can also be terribly inconvenient at times. It can blow up your status quo. Whatever truth can be, there is one thing it always is: Truth is right. I will go one bold step further: **Accepting truth with a growth mindset is *always* right for you.** It is core to SAGe-living.

But the truth is under assault throughout society. Conspiracy theories are peddled to a pliable populace whose grasp on reality gets swept away by the rip current of disinformation. Truth is always maligned when it threatens power or money. Truth is always threatened when lies provide an easier path to gratification.

Your Mischief Mind can even distort the truth. When you hold contradictory positions, such as loving the environment but driving a gas-guzzling car, or wanting to eat a large bowl of buttered popcorn despite having high cholesterol, your Mischief Mind works in overdrive to reconcile the opposing views. Your brain hates cognitive dissonance—holding incompatible beliefs. That gives an opening for your Mischief Mind to contort the truth into twisted logic to ease the mental discomfort. Think about the times when your Mischief Mind created contrived rationalizations for doing things you knew you shouldn't do.

I'll admit that I'm afflicted with cognitive dissonance on occasion. Just now, I was experiencing cognitive dissonance writing about cognitive dissonance. I wish I were making that up. But I'm tired. The words aren't flowing. I thought I'd like to wrap up my morning writing session and look at beautiful art online. My Mischief Mind pleaded its case: *You can't write if you're not inspired. Looking at art will be so relaxing.* But then my SAGe butted in and reminded me that finishing my book is a higher love to me than surfing the internet. I caught myself in the moment and chose to continue writing.

When someone fails to embrace the truth, wrong choices can be made. Values can be compromised. Why would you expect anything different? You need the best information to choose the best response. Just like a judge and jury seek the truth to administer justice, a SAGe seeks the truth to do justice to their well-being. Science can help you with that worthy mission.

Science aims to understand how the world works through experimentation, observation, and analysis. It pursues the unbiased truth. It never uncovers a perfect understanding of our world—natural phenomena are complex, and there are limits to scientific methods and capabilities.

Still, the wave of scientific discovery carries our imperfect, constantly evolving understanding of the world forward. It allows us to apply newfound insights in ways that improve our lives. That's why I placed *science* at the epicenter of the STEER model. I wanted to emphasize the indispensable role science plays in steering you to treat your body, eat, exercise, and rest in a way that optimizes your health (to the extent you can control).

## Optimizing Your Health: Your Lines of Defense

Science and experts should play a vital role in your health. But it all starts with you. **You are your first line of defense in optimizing your health.** As you seek the truth about your health and what actions you should take to get the best results, embrace your responsibility to take care of yourself.

You can begin by acting like an inquisitive scientist. Be mindful of how you feel. Do you have any symptoms of illness? How are your energy levels? Do you notice any concerning changes in your body? Pay attention to the signals your body *sometimes* gives you when something is amiss, and take action to investigate further. Those actions could include more observation, research, or seeing a doctor. But don't procrastinate or fall into the trap of the "ignorance is bliss" mindset. It could cost you your life.

**Health and wellness professionals (the experts) are your second line of defense.** Your commitment to your health will lead you to partner with the big guns—doctors, dietitians, fitness trainers, and other experts—to get much-needed support with assessing your needs and maintaining your health. Not partnering with the experts in health matters is like aspiring to be an Olympic swimmer but shunning the support of coaches and trainers. Optimizing health is a team sport, not a solo endeavor.

A good approach to engaging your second line of defense is establishing a relationship with a primary care provider (PCP). A PCP is a healthcare professional who provides general medical care. A PCP can be your right-hand partner in your lifelong commitment to wellness. They'll create a health profile for you based on your personal and family health history, lifestyle choices, test results, demographics, and current health status. The PCP will then advise you on what preventive and reactive actions you should take to care for your health. The PCP can also diagnose and treat many illnesses directly or refer you to another expert for more specialized needs beyond their general care.

## The Critical Role of Testing

As part of your health strategy, your PCP (and other experts you consult) will recommend how frequently you should be tested and the focus of those tests. Testing helps detect health trends, diagnose medical conditions (some may not show symptoms), and guide treatments. It can catch issues early while they are more treatable. The testing types range from vital sign measurements, physical exams, and blood work to imaging tests, genetic tests, and others.

Testing is a lot of fun. You go to a doctor's office and get poked and prodded. I can't think of a better way to spend an afternoon. Unless you saw a movie of course. That would be more fun. And bowling is enjoyable. I'd rather bowl than get tested. Even picking up dry cleaning—all right, testing is not fun! But testing is critical to ensuring your health approach aligns with your needs.

Let's continue our exploration of the STEER model. Next up is a treat.

## Science – **Treat** – Eat – Exercise – Rest

You can do all the right things to live the healthiest life possible, yet you will become ill in your lifetime. Your body may be a temple, but it's not a Greek temple made of marble that will hold up for thousands of years. It's more like a wooden temple with leaky windows, stained carpet, and an air-conditioning unit on the fritz. I won't mention the termite infestation—that would be too depressing. Don't you just love your body?

Your body is not built to last. Your spirit is, I believe, but not your physical being. Impermanence is the reality for all life forms. A Self-Actualized Genius accepts that truth and does their best with what they can control. And there's a lot you can control. You can be intentional with what you eat, how often you exercise, and how much rest you get. You can be smart with lifestyle choices.

Unfortunately, there's a lot you don't control. You are born with your genetics, both good and bad. Your body wears down as you age. You can get injured in an accident. Disease can occur even if you live a healthy lifestyle. Your health is complex and unpredictable, and despite your best efforts, problems arise. That's why a SAGe seeks treatment to address their medical issues.

But before we discuss the role of treatments, consider the Ben Franklin adage from the 1700s: "An ounce of prevention is worth a pound of cure." With inflation over the centuries, an ounce of prevention is now worth at least seven and a half pounds of cure, but that's splitting hairs. His underlying point is still valid: Preventing bad things is always preferable to suffering through bad things. Preventive care is a vital component of your health strategy.

## Preventive Care

The primary objectives of preventive care are to minimize the risk of illness, enhance overall health, and increase longevity.

Assessing your relationship with toxins is a great place to start when building your strategy. Science and common sense tell you that smoking, vaping, and taking illicit drugs are bad for your health—it's like playing footsies with a rattlesnake. Other toxins, such as alcohol, can also be harmful. If you choose to drink alcohol, drink in moderation. The CDC (Centers for Disease Control and Prevention) defines moderate daily drinking as two drinks or less for men and one drink or less for women.[3] If you struggle with substances, summon your SAGe and seek help (counseling, rehabilitation, tobacco cessation programs). Don't wait. You can't soar if addiction has you tethered to the ground.

Another preventive care strategy is to work with your PCP and determine which vaccines and supplements you should take. Those proactive measures can be crucial gap closers for you and cover health needs that exercise, diet, and rest may fall short of fully addressing. For example, you will likely be exposed to the influenza virus and coronavirus despite your precautions. Fortunately, effective vaccines are available that can greatly lessen the severity of health issues caused by both viruses.

The rest of the components of the STEER model also contribute significantly to preventing illness. Your health—to the level you can control—is a function of science, treat, eat, exercise, and rest, and how they work together. If one of those components is underserved, the weak link can disrupt your entire well-being.

If you are proactive with prevention, you'll increase your odds of good health. But issues will still occur. That brings us to *treatments*.

## Treatments

Stupid happens. You can prevent some stupid sometimes, but stupid will still find a way to happen, for that's what stupid does. Stupid does stupid things in the stupidest ways at the stupidest times. In slightly more articulate words, sometimes you will need medical intervention, no matter how well you care for your body.

Medical intervention comes in many forms, from taking an aspirin to relieve a headache to more advanced treatments like therapy and surgery. Some treatments can be safely administered by you, while others require partnering with the health and wellness community.

In this section, I won't cover specific treatments for specific illnesses— that is well beyond the scope of this book—but I will expand upon partnering with health and wellness professionals. A common mistake is to take a passive role. After all, they're the experts, right? They are, but it is your life. It always serves your interests to be an active partner when you work with an expert.

I'll give an example. During my daughter Emma's vicious odyssey battling headaches, we worked with many terrific experts. But we also dealt with a doctor who doubted whether Emma felt the pain she described. His cynicism angered me. Another doctor had no interest in diagnosing the root cause of her condition. He said we would probably never find out. He simply prescribed pain relief medication. We switched doctors in both cases.

My wife and I quickly learned we needed to be in the driver's seat regarding Emma's health. And in typical fashion, Emma soon relegated us to backseat drivers as she grabbed the steering wheel to navigate her own life.

Following are some principles that helped us forge a productive partnership with health and wellness professionals:

- *Recognize that you are your best health advocate.* Experts care. But they serve many people—they're not thinking about you constantly. You have the benefit of serving one primary person, yourself. Don't settle for anything less than getting the care you need. Be a respectful yet dogged advocate for your health.

- *Trust the experts, but verify.* Research your symptoms and condition. Write down your questions and get them answered when you engage with the pros. Get a second opinion when necessary. Your due diligence will help you make informed health decisions based on the best available information.

- *Evaluate the service you receive and make a change if necessary.* Some experts are better than others. Switch to someone new if the care you receive falls short of what you need. It may take multiple experts to diagnose and treat a complicated medical condition.

- *Control what you can; surrender to what you can't.* Apply the Accept-Frame-Respond model and move forward by choosing your SAGe-inspired, expert-guided response to your health condition.

If you take these common-sense approaches to your partnership with the health and wellness community, you'll put yourself in a position to get better outcomes. But enough talk about treatments—I'm hungry!

## Science – Treat – **Eat** – Exercise – Rest

Kindly channel your inner Paul McCartney and sing along with me:

*Woke up, stayed in bed*
*Purged the thought of exercise from my head*
*Found my way downstairs and slurped an energy drink*
*And looking at my iPhone, I noticed I was late*
*Scarfed my frozen waffles, margarine, and maple goo*
*Made the Uber in seconds flat*
*Found my way to the office and had a doughnut*
*And somebody spoke and I went into a food coma*

Out of my love for the Beatles, I won't parody their classic song "A Day in the Life" anymore. But does that ever describe your morning, or something close to it? In a rush, you skip exercising and then fill your stomach with empty calories, candy, and convenience as you go about your day, oblivious to the health fallout. A healthy start to your morning is essential to your well-being.

Let's explore breakfast options (we'll cover exercise in the next section). Instead of shoveling down the frozen waffles, we could have savored my breakfast ritual of oatmeal cooked with soy milk, blueberries, bananas, flaxseed, and walnuts. It would have only taken a few minutes to prepare.

I'll share the ingredient list for both choices. Note: The ingredient breakdown for the frozen waffle breakfast excludes the doughnut snack mentioned in the song because I don't want you to weep every time you eat fried dough loaded with icing, jellies, creams, and other sinful delights. Though weeping would be a well-reasoned response.

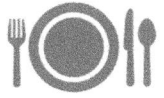 *Breakfast Menu*

## Processed

### FROZEN WAFFLES & THE FIXINS

*Frozen waffles smothered with margarine and gooey artificial maple syrup. Served with a canned energy drink.*

Ingredients

**waffles** (enriched flour, water, vegetable oil, sugar, leavening (baking soda, sodium aluminum phosphate, monocalcium phosphate), salt, dextrose, spice, whey, eggs, soy lecithin, vitamins and minerals), **margarine** (vegetable oil blend, soybean oil, water, buttermilk, salt, potassium sorbate, soy lecithin and mono and diglycerides, lactic acid, natural and artificial flavor, vitamin A palmitate, beta-carotene), **artificial maple syrup** (corn syrup, high fructose corn syrup, water, cellulose gum, caramel color, salt, natural and artificial flavor, sodium benzoate and sorbic acid, sodium hexametaphosphate), **energy drink** (carbonated water, sugar, glucose, citric acid, natural flavors, taurine, sodium citrate, color added, Panax ginseng extract, L-carnitine L-tartrate, caffeine, sorbic acid, benzoic acid, niacinamide, sucralose, salt, D-glucuronolactone, inositol, guarana extract, pyridoxine hydrochloride, riboflavin, maltodextrin, cyanocobalamin)

## Natural

### LOADED ORGANIC OATMEAL

*Oatmeal cooked with soymilk and milled flaxseed and topped with blueberries, walnuts, and bananas. Served with a glass of orange juice.*

Ingredients (all organic)

**oats, soy milk** (water, soybeans, vitamin and mineral blend, sea salt, gellan gum, ascorbic acid, natural flavor), **milled flaxseed, blueberries, walnuts, bananas, orange juice**

The ingredients in the frozen waffle breakfast represent a delicate balance engineered by food manufacturers to create cheap, mass-producible foods that maintain long shelf lives while appealing to a human's craving for fats and sugars. Take a close look at both options. Which option seems healthier, more wholesome? How about tastier?

If you chose the frozen waffle breakfast, are you comfortable eating mysterious ingredients created in a lab and not nature? What do you think about the added sugar, salt, and artificial flavor and color?

Many people eat processed food because it can be cheap and convenient. But, as we'll learn, your body pays a price if it dominates your diet. Every healthy food you eat is a step toward wellness. Is your gut telling you to commit to better nutrition? My SAGe is hollering at me right now to do so!

Healthy eating starts with obtaining nutrition knowledge and is followed by what you do with those insights. Do you know which foods are good for you? And then, do you follow through and choose the healthier foods?

In keeping with the 80/20 rule, I'll provide a baseline of healthy nutritional practices (*Healthy Eating—8 SAGe Tips*) followed by guidance on how you can make them a habitual part of your life (*Healthy Eating—Choose Your Response*). As always, I encourage you to do further research on the topics that interest you and work with experts to customize your approach.

## Healthy Eating—8 SAGe Tips

An argument could be made that your diet impacts your physical health more than any other factor. It would at least be a hearty debate. Your diet provides the essential nutrients—vitamins and minerals, fats, protein, carbohydrates, fiber, and water—that your body needs to function properly. A healthy diet supports physical health, increases energy levels, helps manage weight, and enhances mental health.

An important part of healthy eating is ensuring your diet provides enough energy, measured by calories, to sustain your life. Calories are a standard measurement used to determine the energy content of what you put into your body. If you don't consume enough calories, you'll lack the energy to fully engage in life. If you eat too many, you'll feel sluggish. If overeating leads to being overweight or obese, it can increase the risk of health issues, including heart disease, type 2 diabetes, and certain cancers. There are online resources and experts (dietitians, nutritionists) that can help you set a daily calorie target based on your health needs, demographics, activity levels, and other factors.

If you build healthy eating habits—what you eat, when you eat, and how much you eat—you should get all the nutrition you need without going on a specialized diet or taking supplements. The operative word is *if*. Of course, there are always exceptions to that rule, such as being pregnant, having a nutritional deficiency, training for a sport, or having a medical condition.

To cover the basics of healthy eating practices, here are 8 SAGe Tips:

## SAGe TIP #1: **FULFILL YOUR VITAMIN AND MINERAL NEEDS WITH NUTRIENT-DENSE FOODS**

Eating nutrient-dense foods (high ratio of nutrients to calories) optimizes nutrition and reduces the risk of obesity (a win-win). To bring more nutrient-dense foods into your diet, you can start by reading the nutritional labels of what you eat to understand the levels of vitamins and minerals and other nutrients you get for the calories consumed (if a nutrition label isn't available, check online). That awareness alone can trigger your SAGe to nudge you to choose healthy foods that cover the gamut of your nutritional needs.

Another way to make nutrient density a part of your diet is to eat a "rainbow" of plants daily. Besides providing essential nutrition, plants also contain phytonutrients, which are compounds that give plants color and help protect them against pathogens and insects. Phytonutrients also benefit humans by reducing the risk of many diseases. Each color—red, orange and yellow, green, blue and purple, and white and brown—provides different health benefits.

To illustrate the power of nutrient density and intentional eating, here's a starter list of vitamins and minerals, the benefits they provide, and nutrient-dense food sources. Note: This chart is a small sampling.

| Vitamins and Minerals | 3 Benefits to the Body | Examples of Nutrient-Dense Food Sources |
|---|---|---|
| Vitamin A | vision, immunity, growth and development | carrots, spinach, dairy, sweet potatoes, organ meats |
| Vitamin B9 | cell growth, protein metabolism, blood health | lentils, spinach, asparagus, fortified cereal, Brussels sprouts |
| Vitamin B12 | nerve function, blood health, DNA synthesis | beef liver, salmon, eggs, fortified cereal, dairy |
| Vitamin C | immunity, healing, antioxidant properties | citrus fruits, strawberries, kiwi-fruit, red and green peppers, broccoli |
| Vitamin D | bone and teeth health, muscle function, immunity | fortified dairy, fortified plant-based milk, fortified cereal, fatty fish, sunlight (non-food source) |
| Vitamin E | antioxidant properties, immunity, vision | nuts and seeds, vegetable oils, avocados, salmon, red peppers |
| Calcium | bone and teeth health, nerve function, muscle function | dairy, fortified plant-based milk, fortified cereal, leafy greens, almonds |
| Iron | blood health, immunity, energy metabolism | lean beef and poultry, spinach, lentils, shellfish, fortified cereal |
| Potassium | nerve function, heart function, fluid balance | bananas, oranges, potatoes, apricots, beans |
| Zinc | immunity, growth and development, skin health | shellfish, lean beef and poultry, nuts and seeds, dairy, whole grains |

Have fun buying nutrient-dense foods and experimenting with recipes. If you find a nutrient-dense food unappetizing—no matter how you prepare it—simply drown it with hot sauce. A longitudinal scientific study conducted in my kitchen has shown that hot sauce makes everything taste better.

### SAGe TIP #2: **CHOOSE HEALTHY FATS**

Fats are essential for your health. They provide energy to your body, increase nutrient absorption, protect organs, and serve many other functions. To keep it simple, I'll focus on two types of fats: saturated and unsaturated.

Saturated fats are often solid at room temperature. They come from animal products like meat, eggs, and dairy, and certain oils such as coconut and palm. Saturated fats raise "bad" (LDL) cholesterol levels in the blood, which increases the risk of heart disease and strokes. When eating saturated fats, choose healthier versions, including lean meat, skinless poultry, and low-fat dairy.

Unsaturated fats are considered 'healthy' fats because they help lower LDL cholesterol in the bloodstream while raising "good" (HDL) cholesterol levels. Unsaturated fats are found in nuts and seeds, vegetable oils (extra-virgin olive oil is a healthy fat superstar), avocados, fatty fish, and other foods. Strive to replace saturated fats with unsaturated fats and moderate your fat intake to avoid excess calories.

### SAGe TIP #3: **SEEK PROTEIN-RICH FOODS (PLANT-BASED IS PREFERRED)**

Proteins are essential for nearly every bodily function, including supporting cell growth and muscle development, providing structure to the body, strengthening the immune system, and serving as hormones and enzymes.

Protein is made up of amino acids, which are organic molecules that string together in combinations to form the thousands of proteins we need.

Foods from animal sources generally provide all of the types of amino acids the body requires and are considered complete protein sources. Plant-based foods also provide amino acids, but most are incomplete protein sources (some essential amino acids will be supplied, while others will not). When plants are the primary source of a person's protein, it's important to eat a variety of plants to help ensure that a combination of plants covers the body's amino acid needs.

Eating plant-based protein sources can lower cholesterol, help manage weight, and decrease the risk of early death. According to a Harvard cohort study, healthy eating patterns centered around fruits, vegetables, whole grains, nuts, and legumes (beans, lentils, chickpeas, soybeans, peas, and peanuts) resulted in a 20% lower risk of early death from all causes.[4]

Examples of protein sources include nuts and seeds, legumes (soybeans are a complete protein source), whole grains (quinoa is a complete protein source), artichokes, asparagus, kale, spinach, potatoes, Brussels sprouts, eggs, dairy, fish, shellfish, white meat poultry, and lean beef.

### SAGe TIP #4: **REPLACE SIMPLE CARBS WITH COMPLEX CARBS**

When you eat carbohydrates (carbs)—foods containing sugar, starch, or fiber—your digestive system breaks down the digestible carbs (sugar and starch) and transforms them into glucose, which supplies your body with energy. Fiber is a carb that the body can't digest—see SAGe Tip #5.

Not all carbs are created equal. Complex carbs (starch and fiber) are preferred to simple carbs (sugar). Starch, for example, takes longer to digest than sugar and is converted into glucose more slowly, providing energy to your body over a longer period. Starch also has a much higher nutritional value than sugar and can help with weight control since it is more filling.

Examples of starchy foods include bread, rice, pasta, potatoes, cereals, corn, whole grains, squash, turnips, beans, and lentils.

SAGe TIP #5: **INCLUDE HIGH-FIBER FOODS IN YOUR DIET**

Fiber is a nondigestible component of plant-based foods. A high-fiber diet supports digestive health, helps maintain healthy blood sugar and cholesterol levels, reduces the risk of certain diseases, and assists with weight control by making you feel full longer.

Examples of high-fiber foods include nuts and seeds, whole grains, legumes, and many fruits and vegetables.

SAGe TIP #6: **STAY HYDRATED**

Water serves many vital functions in your body, including eliminating waste, aiding digestion, helping your brain function, preventing dehydration, promoting healthy skin, and regulating body temperature.

Experts differ on how much water a person should drink each day. One common guideline is to drink eight glasses. Another is to drink an ounce of water for every two pounds of body weight. Some experts recommend drinking even more. The right amount for you depends upon your age, weight, and activity levels, the climate, and other factors.

To ensure proper hydration, listen to when your body signals it needs hydration—thirst, sluggishness, muscle cramps, dry mouth, disorientation—and adjust your fluid intake accordingly. Consider keeping water by your side wherever you are to encourage frequent hydration.

SAGe TIP #7: **CHOOSE WHOLE AND ORGANIC FOODS (WHENEVER POSSIBLE)**

Whole foods are natural, unprocessed foods free from additives and artificial ingredients. When food is processed, unhealthy ingredients like saturated fats, sugar, and excessive salt are often added, and industrial processing methods (heating, milling, refining) can strip nutrients from the food.

Organic foods are free from synthetic pesticides and fertilizers, antibiotics, hormones, artificial preservatives, and other unnatural modifications.

There are significant health benefits associated with whole and organic foods. Two studies published in the *British Medical Journal* in 2019 showed that people who eat less ultra-processed food (manufactured food that contains minimal whole ingredients) have a lower risk of heart disease, manage weight better, and live longer.[5] Other studies have shown that nonorganic foods can have a lower nutritional value than their organic counterparts and may contribute to Alzheimer's disease and a host of other health issues (due to pesticide exposure).[6]

### SAGe TIP #8: **BALANCE YOUR NUTRITION**

A healthy, balanced diet is generally rich in a diverse selection of whole grains, fruits, vegetables, lean proteins, and healthy fats. Most daily diets include three meals and one or two snacks. The timing of your food intake is important to your energy levels. To stay alert, glucose (which comes from carbs) should be replenished at regular intervals, usually every three or four hours. Your body signals when it's hungry—be on the lookout for low energy, poor concentration, shakiness, headaches, irritability, and the telltale growling stomach.

A guideline for meal portion control is to fill half of your plate with fruits and vegetables (more veggies than fruit due to their lower sugar content), one-quarter with grains (whole grains are healthier due to less processing), and one-quarter with protein (plant-based is healthier, but avoid ultra-processed versions). A serving of dairy or a fortified dairy substitute should also be included.[7] For snacks, choose healthy options, such as an apple with nut butter, carrots, hummus and veggies, edamame, and fruit and veggie smoothies.

Now that you have actionable insights about nutrition and how it can improve your well-being, let's put that knowledge to use!

## Healthy Eating—Choose Your Response

Healthy eating provides the essential nourishment to sustain your healthiest life possible. When you follow a healthy diet aligned with your values, you nurture the wonderful gift of your existence.

A key to performing well with nutrition is translating your knowledge about healthy eating into guidelines you follow. Make healthy eating an inseparable part of your identity. Be a SAGe who chooses diverse, nutrient-dense foods that cover your nutritional needs. Control your portions. Stay well-hydrated. Moderate your indulgences.

If you do stuff like that, you probably won't need to count calories or fret over a perfect nutritional balance for every meal, unless you have health reasons to do so. Healthy eating will happen naturally because it's what you do; it's who you are. Getting to that point requires changing behaviors and building habits, meal by meal. As we know, the good things in life are rarely spoon-fed to us, so planning and commitment are also part of the success equation.

A straightforward process, patterned after the change adoption process we covered in chapter 6 (Why? – Define – Position – Do), can help you get on a good path with your diet (if you're not already there). Let's work through that.

### WHY? – DEFINE – POSITION – DO

Why do you want to focus on healthy eating? How will it support your life purpose and quality of life? Does it impact your family? Connect with your why and let it motivate and inspire you.

Your why could center around wanting to feel good and have the energy to pursue your passions. You could be focused on living longer or setting an inspiring example for your children. The stronger your why, the more likely you'll adopt healthy habits.

If you struggle to feel motivated to focus on your health, whether it's healthy eating, exercising, or another aspect, meditate on it and envision what it would be like to be a model of healthy living. What are you doing? How are you feeling as you go about your day? How is your self-esteem? Is there a spiritual purpose to healthy living? Connect with wellness at a deeper, more personal level—make it real. Let that inspire you to find a why you believe in.

### WHY? – **DEFINE** – POSITION – DO

Before you fire away and develop objectives and a plan to realize them, you'll want to ensure you're aiming at the right target. Start with your baseline. You probably have both healthy and unhealthy eating habits. You may have a diet relying on processed foods. You could have high cholesterol or be overweight. To determine where you're at and what your needs are, factor in:

○  *How do you feel?* How are your energy levels throughout the day?

○  *What does the science tell you?* What are your medical test results? Do you have health issues? Nutritional gaps? What do the experts think? If you haven't had tests recently, consider scheduling them.

○  *Do you have specialized needs?* Are you an athlete? Are you pregnant? Do you have food allergies? Are there special considerations that should be factored into your approach to healthy eating?

○  *What are your dietary habits, and are they covering your nutritional needs?* There are many ways to assess that. You could keep a food diary and record the calories and nutrients you consume for a week to see how you perform compared to dietary guidelines. A more effective approach would be to track it on an app. Diet and fitness apps are easy to use (some are free), and they'll do the nutritional analysis for you.

From your baseline analysis and the perspective of experts, how can your diet serve you? Improve your health? Close nutritional gaps? Lose weight? Increase energy? Lower cholesterol? Build muscle? All of the above?

Examples of objectives could include reducing the consumption of ultra-processed foods by 30%, trying a new nutrient-dense food each week and incorporating the ones you like into your regular diet, lowering daily caloric intake to a healthy range, and adhering to a balanced, nutritious diet.

### WHY? – DEFINE – **POSITION** – DO

Once you have established your objectives, the next step is to develop a plan to make them real. What will you do specifically with your diet to achieve your intentions? What is your change adoption approach? The criticality and challenge of your objectives should drive your planning effort. For instance, if you want to improve your energy levels, you will likely need a well-thought-out plan that considers limiting sugar and processed foods; eating smaller, more frequent meals; staying hydrated; preparing balanced meals high in protein, B vitamins, and iron; and incorporating other health strategies, such as exercising, improving sleep, and reducing stress.

There are many approaches to becoming a healthy eater, most of which can be combined. Following are some of the more effective ones:

○ *Work with a dietitian or a nutritionist to customize a dietary approach based on your needs.* Expert support can be the difference between success and failure, especially for challenging objectives.

○ *Leverage a wellness app.* There are apps that can help you plan your wellness approach (diet, exercise, rest, etc.) to meet your health objectives. Apps can track nutrition, calories, exercise, weight, and other factors to help you stay on track. The best ones also offer gamification, nudging, and educational features that increase your odds of success.

○ *Follow an established diet, such as the Mediterranean diet, the DASH diet, or others.* Diets provide a prescriptive approach to nutrition.

But work with an expert to ensure you choose the right one for your needs.

○ *Subscribe to a meal delivery service.* These services help you plan nutritious and portion-controlled meals. They also offer convenience.

○ *Do-it-yourself.* Use the nutritional guidelines detailed in this chapter (add more that resonate) and utilize change adoption techniques to make healthy eating a habit. You could: (1) gamify healthy eating by tracking a healthy eating streak on a calendar, (2) align support by rallying your family or friends to go on a shared journey toward healthier eating, (3) be audacious with your accountability by establishing a motivating reward (or penalty) for your intentions, and (4) anticipate your derailers by ordering groceries online and having healthy snacks available.

The best plans are realistic and aligned with your needs. There are plenty of resources and change adoption techniques at your disposal that can help you be successful. Your health is always worth the effort.

## WHY? – DEFINE – POSITION – **DO**

If your diet doesn't support a healthy lifestyle, changing that can be one of the most challenging transitions you undertake. It often requires replacing deeply ingrained bad habits with good habits. But once you head down a healthy path, you build momentum and confidence. Good habits form. Prioritizing health becomes second nature. In fact, you won't feel right if you slip back into your old ways. Try these practices to ease your transition to healthy eating:

○ *Practice mindful eating.* Enjoy the moment of eating a delicious, healthy meal. Savor every bite. Think about the nutrition being absorbed by your body and nourishing your cells. According to science, slow eaters tend to be less obese than fast eaters.[8]

○ *Repeat the mantra: "I am a healthy eater. I am a healthy eater."* Remind yourself of your commitment to healthy eating throughout the day. Soon, you'll believe it and strive for better nutrition.

○ *Eat until you're satisfied, not until you're full.* Don't feel obligated to finish everything on your plate—stop when satisfied. You can also practice "one less" to teach yourself portion control. Remind yourself to take "one less" of what you typically eat. Take one less serving of meat, one less scoop of ice cream, or one less spoonful of potatoes. You'll develop the habit of eating what your body needs, not what your Mischief Mind craves.

○ *Drink a glass or two of water before a meal to control overeating.* The water will fill your stomach, making you less hungry. It will also help with digestion.

○ *Allow for reasonable indulgences.* Some foods have limited nutritional value but are so damn good. Vanilla milkshakes and french fries are my kryptonite. Life is better when I'm eating them, but my life would be short-lived if I ate them whenever I wanted to, which would be hourly. So I allow myself a cheat day once a week. That approach controls my cravings since I know there's a time set aside to indulge.

○ *Front-load calories to breakfast and lunch.* Doing so ensures you have enough nutrients and energy to engage in the day. Consuming food at night aids overnight metabolic processes, so don't skip dinner, but avoid overindulging since fewer calories are needed in the evening.

○ *Make it your mission to experiment with healthy recipes.* Have fun finding and cooking healthy recipes with your family. Rate the meals when you're done. Keep track of the ones you like.

○ *Substitute healthy food for less healthy food.* Fruit for candy, brown rice for white rice, water for soda, nonfat Greek yogurt for sour cream, nuts for chips . . . Every healthy substitution is a gift to your body.

How do you respond when you're in the moment of truth—in a grocery store deciding what to buy, at home determining what to eat, or in a restaurant choosing what to order? Do you make healthy choices to respect your body? It is always within your capability to do so. You can make healthy eating a habit. You do it choice by choice, meal by meal.

Eating healthy is a lifelong commitment. If you stumble (we all do), learn from your experience, reestablish your footing, and move forward. Seek help if necessary. *Don't give up.* You have too much riding on it.

Are you ready to burn some calories?

## Science – Treat – Eat – **Exercise** – Rest

You were built to move. When you exert yourself, your heart beats faster. Your lungs work harder. Your brain perks up. You feel better (you can thank the endorphin surge for that).

After you exercise, the good feeling carries forward. Different exercises affect you in different ways. But think about this: Have you ever regretted going for a walk? Has it ever failed to lift your spirits and energize you?

Science also supports the benefits of exercise. A comprehensive scientific review of cohort studies showed that lifespan increased by a range of 0.4 to 6.9 additional years for physically active people compared to inactive people.[9] Or look at exercise and mental health. According to a Yale study, "Individuals who exercised had 43.2% fewer days of poor mental health in the past month than individuals who did not exercise."[10]

Exercise comes in a thousand forms, including jogging, walking, hiking, yoga, swimming, bike riding, dancing, sheep herding, weightlifting, and countless others. Your approach to exercise—how often and which types—should depend upon your health profile, objectives, and how your body responds to the physical activity. A fitness expert can help you sort through the best exercise routines based on your needs.

For the Wellness Ethic, I'll offer an 80/20 perspective on the essentials of fitness, with a focus on three types of exercise:

○ *Mobility*: exercises that improve the range of motion and flexibility of your joints and muscles

○ *Cardiorespiratory*: exercises that increase your heart and breathing rates

○ *Strength*: exercises that maintain and build muscle mass

By incorporating all three exercises into your weekly routines, you'll put yourself in a better position to live a healthy life. But before I explore each exercise type, I'll provide a very important level set: Don't expect to see shirtless pictures of me showcasing my one-pack abs as I demonstrate proper techniques for recommended exercises. The images would go viral and destabilize the world order.

## Mobility Exercise

*Mobility* is defined as the ability of a joint and accompanying muscles to engage in a full range of motion. Improving your mobility can lower your risk of injuries, relieve aches and stiffness, elevate workout and athletic performance, and improve your posture. Mobility is also vital to a person's ability to effortlessly perform everyday tasks, like bending down to pick up something, and can impact their ability to be independent (especially as they age).

There are many types of mobility exercises. An internet search will provide hundreds of examples—with pictures and videos—that can be targeted to specific joint and muscle groups. Two common types of mobility exercises are dynamic stretching, which are movements that take your joints and muscles through their full range of motion, and static stretching, which involves holding a stretch to lengthen muscles and increase flexibility.

How frequently you should do mobility exercises, and for what duration, depends upon your objectives and the results you attain. A general guideline is to perform mobility exercises at least two to three times a week for ten to thirty minutes per session. Spreading your mobility exercises throughout the week, rather than doing them all at once, is more effective.

An easy way to establish a mobility exercise habit is to include mobility exercises before a cardiorespiratory or strength workout, targeting the muscles and joints you plan to use. By doing so, you'll prepare your body for the stress of the workout, which can lead to better performance and lower injury risk. And by stacking the mobility exercise habit with another exercise habit, you're more likely to remember to complete your mobility routine. Another effective approach is to do mobility exercises first thing in the morning or before bed.

## Cardiorespiratory Exercise

Cardiorespiratory exercise—also known as cardiovascular (cardio) or aerobic exercise—is a type of physical activity that elevates your heart and breathing rates by repeatedly moving large muscle groups over a sustained period. The benefits are profound and include lowering the risk of many diseases, managing weight, increasing stamina, bolstering immunity, increasing life expectancy, and improving mood and brain function.[11]

To establish our baseline standards, I'll shamelessly borrow from the experts. The US Department of Health and Human Services (HHS), in their *Physical Activity Guidelines for Americans—2nd Edition*, established aerobic activity guidelines for adults. Here are a few of the essential standards:

○ Increase movement and decrease sitting throughout the day.

○ Spread physical activity throughout the week.

○ Target at least 150 minutes of *moderate-intensity* physical activity per week (which can translate to 30 minutes a day, 5 days a week).[12]

Moderate-intensity activities include walking briskly, bike riding, water aerobics, recreational swimming, mowing, doubles tennis, in-line skating, and other activities that elevate your heart and breathing rates.

So, how much is enough, and should you include higher-intensity exercises like jogging, running on a treadmill, or rowing? Your age, gender, health profile, and fitness objectives all play a role in determining your best approach. I'll defer to you and the experts to determine your plan.

## COUNTING STEPS

Counting steps is a popular approach to ensuring you stay active. *Gotta get my 10,000 steps in!* How many times have you heard something like that? You see people on a virtual team meeting bouncing up and down as they walk on a treadmill, or constantly checking their devices to see how many steps they've recorded for the day. They're participating in one of the best examples of gamification on the planet—counting the number of steps you take on an app as you march toward your daily step target.

The concept of counting 10,000 steps per day originated from a 1960s Japanese marketing campaign for a pedometer, and it became the conventional wisdom exercise target for healthy living. However, a recent cohort study published in 2021 determined that people who took just 7,000 steps or more per day had a 50% to 70% lower mortality risk than those who took fewer than 7,000 steps.[13]

So, should you target 7,000 steps a day? That's a healthy intention. You may also consider increasing your daily step target to achieve other benefits, such as weight loss or weight maintenance.

I like the concept of counting steps. It promotes being active throughout the day. Many smartphones and apps can count the steps for you, so tracking is easy as you move about, and their gamification features can be motivating. Soon, you'll park farther away from a store to get more steps in. You'll take the stairs instead of an elevator. You'll find creative ways to keep your steps streak alive.

Developing a cardiorespiratory exercise habit requires intentionality. One of the best ways to adopt the practice is to make it a part of your morning or early evening routines. That way, you know you'll exercise at a particular time each day. You don't have to think about it. It's just what you do.

Chapter 6 offers other best practices to help you develop an exercise habit. Aligning the support of a fitness expert or an exercise buddy is effective. Creating an instigation habit by setting out your workout clothes the night prior can work. Or consider setting up a motivating reward.

## Strength Exercise

Most adults neglect regular strength exercises. However, incorporating them into your weekly routines can increase your metabolism, improve your strength and flexibility, reduce the risk of injury, improve bone health, and even help you live longer.

To bring science into the mix (because that's what I do!), I'll share a compelling study: A meta-analysis published in the *British Journal of Sports Medicine* showed that performing just thirty to sixty minutes of muscle-strengthening activities per week was "associated with a 10–17% lower risk of all-cause mortality."[14]

Strength training can consist of lifting barbells and kettlebells (or even water jugs), using your body weight as resistance (push-ups, pull-ups), doing chores such as chopping wood, exercising with resistance bands, or using advanced exercise equipment. Your routine can be straightforward if you want to attain the core health benefits of strength training, or it can be more involved if you are training for a sport, rehabbing, or striving for peak performance.

Consider these steps when starting a strength-building routine (in consultation with a fitness expert):

○ *Step 1: Set your objectives.* Do you want to establish a basic routine or strive for more? Do you want to build muscle for strength, endurance, or both? Strength exercises involve fewer reps with more resistance; endurance exercises include more reps and less resistance.

○ *Step 2: Select your exercise location and equipment (if any).* Do you want to get a gym membership or work out at home? Do you want to use barbells, kettlebells, resistance bands, free weights, or other equipment? What about using your body weight? You don't need expensive equipment to achieve a great workout.

○ *Step 3: Design your workout session.* Determine your exercises, resistance levels, and reps—many free online routines exist Your chosen exercises should cover your major muscle groups.

○ *Step 4: Establish your strength-building weekly routine.* Typically, you should do strength exercises two or three times a week for at least twenty to thirty minutes a session, but your needs could vary from that norm. As you plan your schedule, include at least one off-day between sessions to give your muscles time to recover from the workout.

○ *Step 5: Determine your change adoption strategy.* Do you want to set a reward to motivate yourself to adopt the strength-building habit? Or work out with a friend to boost accountability? Tracking an exercise streak on an app or a calendar is also effective.

As with most novel activities, keeping it simple initially helps you build a habit. Get your body used to the training. Don't push yourself too far as you learn the proper form and understand your limitations. You'll build up to more efficient and effective routines over time. The most important objective is to establish a safe exercise habit that stands the test of time.

## What to Do Before, During, and After a Workout

When you exercise, you expend energy, stretch and stress your muscles, and lose water through sweating and respiration.

*Before your workout*, prepare your body for performance. Consider starting with mobility exercises targeting the muscles you plan to use. This increases blood flow to your muscles and loosens joints, reducing the risk of injury. Drink water to ensure you're well hydrated. Eating carbs provides your body with energy, while eating protein benefits muscle repair.

If the workout is expected to last longer than sixty minutes, consuming electrolytes is beneficial since they can be lost through sweat. Electrolytes are minerals—sodium, potassium, magnesium, calcium, chloride, phosphate, and bicarbonate—that aid in bodily functions. Many sports drinks or foods, such as bananas, chocolate milk, oranges, and yogurt, are good electrolyte sources.

Choosing to eat before exercising, and how far in advance, should be influenced by the intensity and duration of the workout, how long it will take for the food to digest, and your body's response.

*During your workout*, it's important to stay hydrated. If the workout will exceed sixty minutes, consider replenishing electrolytes and eating simple carbs (for quick energy) as you exercise.

*After your workout*, the primary objective is to help your body recover. Cooling down with static stretching can prevent stiffness. Rehydrating replaces fluids lost during exercise. Refueling your body with a snack containing protein and carbs aids muscle recovery and restores energy. Replenishing electrolytes (if you had a long or sweaty workout) restores electrolyte balance and supports rehydration and muscle recovery.

## Developing an Exercise Routine

Starting an exercise regimen that covers the three exercise types doesn't have to be overwhelming. You can pick one exercise, start small, and focus on establishing a daily routine—even if that routine lasts just five minutes. You can build upon the routine over time, exercise by exercise.

I'll share what has been effective for me. I've established a set time that I exercise—I wake up at 4:00 a.m. (early to bed, early to rise) and begin working out at 4:30. Following is my weekly routine:

| Sun | Mon | Tue | Wed | Thu | Fri | Sat |
|------|----------|----------|----------|----------|----------|------|
| walk | walk mobility strength | walk mobility treadmill | walk mobility strength | walk mobility treadmill | walk mobility strength | walk |

I start each day by going on a four-mile brisk walk around my neighborhood (8,000 steps). Usually, I walk in silence, enjoy nature, and let my creative mind wander. I do mobility exercises for ten minutes each weekday. For a higher-intensity cardio workout, I use a treadmill twice a week (twenty minutes of brisk walking at 4.3 mph on a 7% incline). For strength training, I use barbells and kettlebells in a twenty-minute routine three times a week.

By completing my exercise habit, I start each day energized and feeling positive. Combine that with my healthy oatmeal breakfast routine, and I'm putting myself in the best position to have a happy and productive day.

We've covered a lot in this section. Reading about exercising is exhausting. It's time to rest.

## Science – Treat – Eat – Exercise – **Rest**

I can't control my sleep patterns, and that irks me. I'd love to hop into bed at 8:00 p.m., shut my eyes, and experience peaceful, bear-like hibernation. In my dream scenario, I'd fall asleep once I hit the sack and wake up seven or eight hours later, bright-eyed and ready to seize the day. If I could reliably get that much uninterrupted sleep each night, my life would be transformed.

But nooooooo! I often fight with my racing mind before falling asleep; sometimes it takes an hour. If the thought of discomfort enters my brain, I obsess over it until I give up and roll over. This overly dramatic process can include a loud sigh, and, at times, the covers get pulled off my wife (regrettably, I maintain). I have learned that such actions result in painful retribution.

My problems don't end there. Most nights, I wake up once or twice to go to the restroom (old age, argh!). Or I must deal with needy cats who don't understand that animals aren't supposed to walk on other animals, especially when the other animals are trying to partake in peaceful, bear-like hibernation!

I need to improve my sleep.

At the risk of providing too much information, the following gives a glimpse into the science behind sleep. If reading it bores you and makes you fall asleep, well, it looks like you have discovered an effective sleep aid!

A sleep cycle consists of three stages of NREM (non-rapid eye movement) sleep and one stage of REM (rapid eye movement) sleep. Most people go through four to six sleep cycles per night, each lasting about 90 to 120 minutes.

As you progress through the NREM stages, your heart and respiration rates decrease, your muscles relax, and your brain wave activity slows. During this time, your body restores itself and strengthens its immune system. The REM sleep stage is characterized by increased heart and respiration rates and rapid eye movements. This stage is when dreaming occurs. REM sleep is important for cognitive brain function, emotional regulation, and memory consolidation.

Getting enough sleep is essential to healthy living. You can exercise, eat well, and work with your doctors to stay healthy, but if you don't get enough sleep, your health and ability to function throughout the day will suffer.

Sleep improves brain function, strengthens your immune system, reduces the risk of heart disease, improves mood, helps with weight control, and increases productivity during waking hours, along with other benefits.[15]

A SAGe needs a healthy amount of sleep to behave like a SAGe. A benchmark sleep target for adults is seven to eight hours a night, though some may need more or less. But achieving perfect sleep every night is an unrealistic expectation—too many variables are out of your control.

However, improving the quality of your sleep is a worthy pursuit. There are many considerations to factor in, and a lot of experimentation will probably need to occur. But every step forward with your sleep will improve the quality of your life. Here are six sleep practices that can help:

○ *Avoid sleep inhibitors.* Some habits impair your ability to sleep, such as consuming caffeine, alcohol, or nicotine in the evening (or even in the afternoon), taking a long nap or a nap later in the afternoon, going to bed hungry or after overeating, and using electronic devices close to bedtime (devices are mentally stimulating, and blue light can suppress melatonin production, which regulates sleep-wake cycles).

○ *Establish a sleep pattern and ritual.* Go to bed at the same time every night. Your body will adjust to the schedule and recognize when it's time to start feeling tired. As part of your routine, clear your mind of stressors—practice meditation or yoga, read, or take an Epsom salt bath. Then, wake up at a consistent time to help regulate your body's internal clock (circadian rhythm). By doing so, you'll feel more refreshed in the morning, and you'll find it easier to fall asleep at night.

○ *Experiment with the tools and techniques of the sleep trade.* What room temperature and level of darkness work best for you? What about your pillows, blankets, and mattress? Should you experiment to see if a change will improve your sleep? Have you tried sleep apps? Or gadgets like a cooling headband, an aroma diffuser (lavender and chamomile can be helpful), a white noise machine, or an eye mask? As you experiment, consider tracking your results in a sleep journal.

- *Have a plan B.* What options do you have if you can't fall asleep? You could try sleeping in another room. The change in scenery could help. Or drink a cup of chamomile tea or a warm glass of milk. Reading a book until you feel drowsy can be effective. Sleep supplements, such as melatonin, are an option, but first consult with a doctor to ensure you avoid adverse drug interactions and other potential risks.

- *Consider well-timed naps and de-stressing activities as part of your rest strategy.* A short, early afternoon nap when tired can help you feel recharged. It can also relieve stress. The same benefits apply to de-stressing activities that you do during the day, such as walking, practicing yoga, and meditating.

- *Seek medical help when necessary.* If poor sleep plagues you, bring it up with your PCP. They may suggest simple remedies, or you may have a sleep disorder requiring specialized attention.

As you work on improving the quality of your sleep, remember to be patient as you embrace experimentation. Accept that perfection will elude you like it eludes billions of other humans. But you can move toward better sleep. And when you do, practically all aspects of your life will improve. Sleep is that important to your well-being.

o o o

## Move Forward on Your Wellness Ethic Journey!

(1) So, how do you feel about what you've learned in this "body" chapter? Do you have enough insights to move forward? Do you feel confident? Let's test your readiness with a pop quiz! Please don't groan. It's unbecoming.

 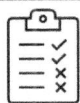

## Pop Quiz

Which of the following activities are considered "approved" forms of exercise by the Wellness Ethic?

A. Lifting your favorite beverage as you watch professionals exercise on TV

B. Stretching to pick up the remote control that dropped to the floor when you reached for your favorite beverage while watching professionals exercise on TV

C. Going for a thirty-minute bike ride around your neighborhood

D. Walking to the fridge so you can grab a snack of organic carrots

### Answer Key

*A: Lifting your favorite beverage as you watch professionals exercise on TV*
Incorrect. Lifting a beverage is a purposeful movement, but you can't forget that there also needs to be a respectable level of physical exertion for the activity to be considered exercise.

*B: Stretching to pick up the remote control that dropped to the floor when you reached for your favorite beverage while watching professionals exercise on TV*
Incorrect. The Wellness Ethic Exercise Rules Committee (WEERC) would have given you exercise credit if you held the stretch for thirty seconds and then repeated the "drop remote control and stretch for thirty seconds" sequence three more times.

*C: Going for a thirty-minute bike ride around your neighborhood*
Correct. You moved! You exerted! Yes!

*D: Walking to the fridge so you can grab a snack of organic carrots*
Incorrect. You walked to the fridge to get the organic carrots. Good snack choice. You should be commended. And walking can often be considered exercise. But WEERC assumed your fridge wasn't across town, so the physical exertion was very limited. You're not getting exercise credit for this.

② Document your intentions for healthy living. If an element of the STEER model is a low priority (because you already have it covered), you can leave it blank. Whatever you decide to move forward with, be sure to apply change adoption techniques as appropriate.

| | Improvement & Change Adoption Focus |
|---|---|
| Science | |
| Treat | |
| Eat | |
| Exercise | |
| Rest | |

③ Advanced Topics (going beyond the 80/20): Research "antioxidants," "omega-3 fatty acids," "intermittent fasting," and "probiotics" to see if there are any healthy practices you want to introduce into your life.

# Mark's Example

(1) Mark passed the pop quiz, on the fourth try, with the help of artificial intelligence.

(2) Document your intentions for healthy living. If an element of the STEER model is a low priority (because you already have it covered), you can leave it blank.

| | Improvement & Change Adoption Focus |
|---|---|
| Science | Continue with annual exams and tests to ensure my approach to physical wellness aligns with my needs. |
| Treat | Continue to take recommended vaccines in consultation with my doctor. |
| Eat | My intentions with my diet are:<br><br>- Eat more nutrient-dense foods.<br><br>- Get my cholesterol down to a healthy range by the end of the year (without using medication).<br><br>- Eat fewer animal-based foods.<br><br>- Savor each wholesome meal and feel grateful for having healthy food on my table.<br><br>Change adoption approach: I'll list these intentions on a piece of paper and tape them to my computer monitor stand as a form of visual management. |
| Exercise | Continue with my weekly exercise habit. It's working! |
| Rest | Experiment with evening de-stressing. |

# Intermission

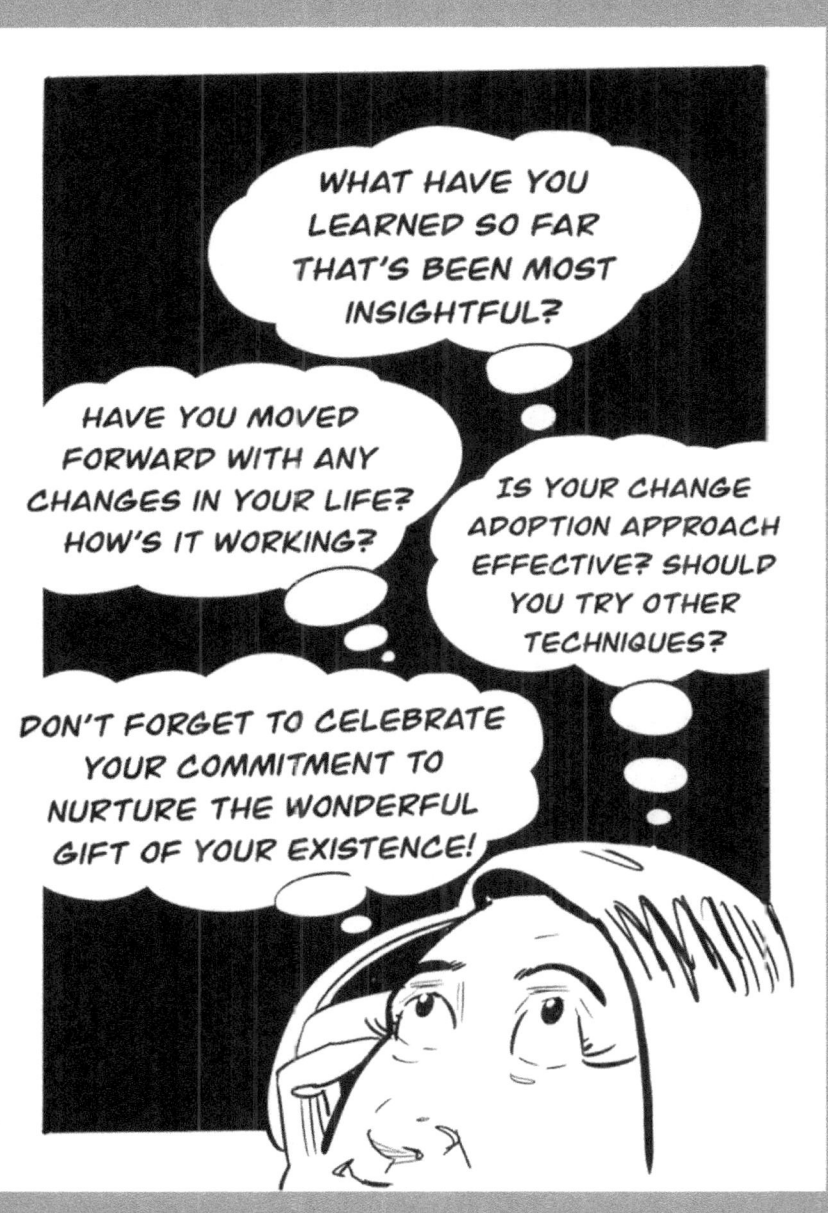

# Relationships

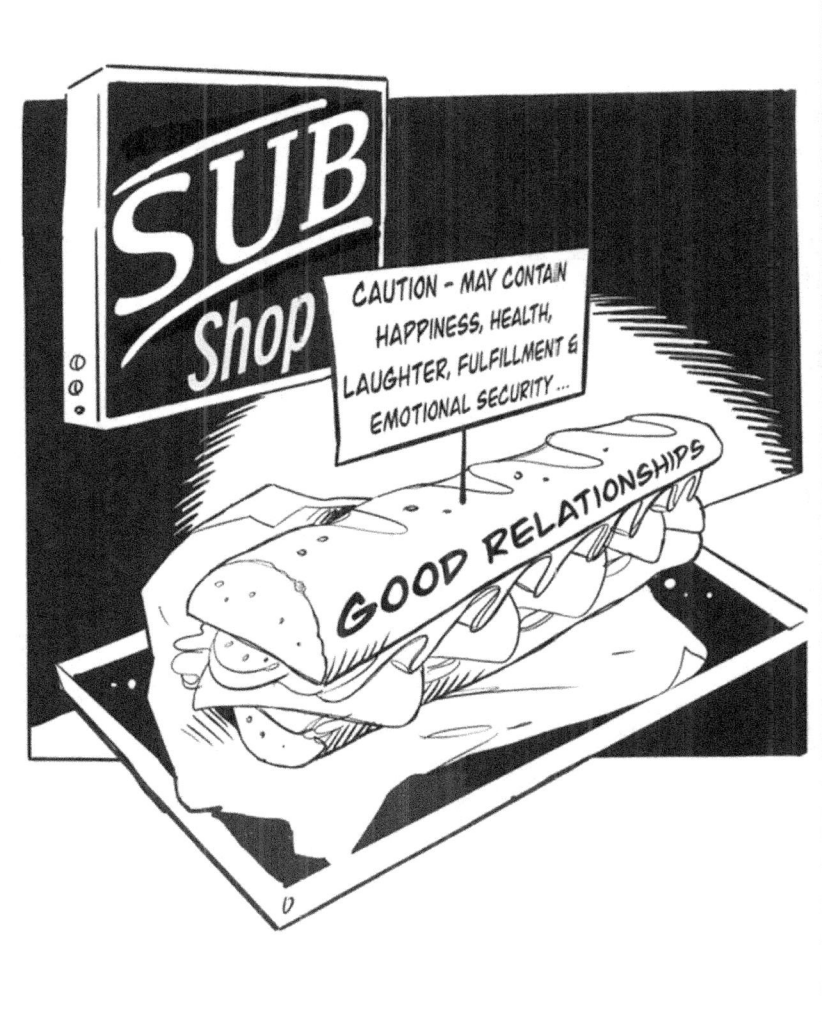

# CHAPTER 13

# A Story of Love

I don't know what possessed me. Over thirty years later, I'm no closer to solving my life's most perplexing mystery.

*What was that Reinisch bloke thinking on November 6, 1992?*

Three ticks of the clock. And then an ordinary Friday night got turned on its head and forever changed two lives. One Mississippi. Two Mississippi. Three Mississippi. My mind raced like a greyhound chasing a rabbit dipped in gravy, but my spirit was calm. Why was that?

I've always been fascinated by *what if*. What if I had moved to Hollywood after college and tried to make it as a screenwriter? What if I left corporate America and became a minister? A life coach? A writer? What if I could make myself invisible? For what it's worth, if the power of invisibility were ever bestowed upon me, I would be very grateful because I think about it a lot. I would also immediately launch my meticulously vetted *Holy Crap! I Can't Believe I Just Became Invisible!* thirty-day plan. I won't share the plan's details here because successful execution relies upon the element of surprise.

Sometimes, my *what-if* contemplations center around happenstance and what if the ball bounced in a different direction during pivotal life moments. My mind is forever teased with the "choose your own adventure" possibilities. Happenstance is where this story begins . . .

It was the spring of 1992. I was in my early twenties and one science elective shy of graduating from Rensselaer Polytechnic Institute (RPI), an engineering university in Troy, New York. To complete my degree, I planned to save money by taking a summer science course at a community college.

But first, I had to find a class. I dropped by Hudson Valley Community College and spoke with an admissions officer. She spent thirty minutes with me examining classes and schedules to see if anything aligned with what I needed. She didn't find anything, so I thanked her and went on my way.

I walked fifteen feet down the hallway, heading for the elevators, when I heard the admissions officer's faint voice: *Mark.*

I continued my stride. *I probably should walk back to see what she wanted. No. There aren't any classes available. I'll figure out something for the fall.* I reached the elevator and was about to press the down button. *Ugh, what the hell?* I walked back to her office. She had found an evening chemistry course that had seating capacity. I looked at the course description; it was promising.

I took the course write-up to RPI, got their transfer approval, and enrolled. That class was where I met my wife, Kristen. It blows my mind that I came so close to not walking back to the admissions officer when she called my name. One simple decision had such far-reaching consequences.

What tugged me to go back? Curiosity? No—I had given up hope that a suitable class was available. Common courtesy? No—I was going to pretend that I didn't hear her. The universe? I've always thought so. You see, at the time, it had been years since I dated. My mind was an echo chamber of limiting beliefs, flatlining my self-esteem. I genuinely believed no one would want to be in a relationship with me. The universe saw it differently.

The courtship of Miss Kristen has been described by scholars as a clumsy affair. Kristen was my lab partner. I was interested in her. She didn't appear to find me repulsive when we worked on our lab assignments, so things were off to a smashing start! But what was I supposed to do? Ask her if she wanted to grab dinner and a movie? I guess I could have done that if

I wanted to go about it like an amateur. But that wasn't the way I wooed romance into my life.

Regarding matters of the heart, I played three-dimensional chess while everyone else played checkers. My plan—and I'd suggest you take notes if you want to be a player like me—was to slow-walk the pursuit and see if my social awkwardness would grow on her over time. Then maybe she'd cave in out of pity and ask me to go on a date. I hadn't succeeded with that plan in the past, but I was confident that my high failure rate reflected my substandard execution rather than the plan itself, which seemed sound to me.

As the summer days plodded on, a casual observer unfamiliar with my plan would have thought I was a buffoon. I imagine someone who walked into class each day lugging an electric fan because the room was sweltering could be perceived as such, especially when they didn't put the fan on oscillating mode so others could enjoy the cool breeze (not my finest hour as a human).

Or when I finished my lab assignment before Kristen, which was always, and pretended to shuffle papers for fifteen awkward minutes rather than just leaving. I wanted to spend time with her without revealing my intentions. It had the opposite effect and led her to believe I was interested in romance—it was painfully obvious—but she thought I was interested in another person in our lab group, a married mother twenty years our senior. I must have sent very confusing signals.

But after about a month, my well-conceived plan paid off. Kristen finally took the initiative to ask me out, kind of—well, not really. She asked a group of students if anyone knew of a sub shop nearby. I suggested Mr. Subb. It piqued her interest. I told her Mr. Subb was on my way home and she could follow me in her car to get there. Kristen was game.

We left class. I drove in my car; she tailed behind. Mr. Subb was about twenty minutes away, and every one of those twenty minutes was filled with overthinking and panic. *What do I do when I get to Mr. Subb?* These were the options I considered:

*I could slow down as I approach Mr. Subb and point at it before driving on.* I would have fulfilled my obligation of getting her to a respectable sandwich purveyor. Any reasonable person would give me credit for that. Hopefully, Kristen was reasonable. This could be a good test of that.

*I could park at Mr. Subb, ensure she safely gets to the door, and then wave to her as I drive away.* It would be chivalrous of me to take that extra step since it was nighttime, and that fact would surely score bonus points. Better yet, by not entering the sub shop with her, I wouldn't risk revealing my romantic interest. That was critical if I wanted to stick to my plan to slow-walk things, which I did because the plan was well thought out.

*I could enter Mr. Subb with her, order a sub for myself, and then leave, whether she sits down to consume her sub or not.* If I entered the sub shop with her, would I be expected to pay her bill? What if I paid for her meal and offended her, or didn't pay for her meal and offended her? Could I strike a balance and offer to pay for her chips and soda but draw the line and ask her to foot the bill for her sub? I knew that idea was a keeper. But what if she sat down and I bolted? That would be perceived as a strange move. Such odd behavior could hinder my chances of dating her, which my plan forecasted to be sometime after I started to collect Social Security in forty years.

*I could enter Mr. Subb with her and ask if she wants to sit down and eat our subs together.* That would be a dumb idea. Way too risky. She would know I was interested, but what if she wasn't? Besides, if she did sit down with me, I would have to engage in small talk, which wasn't a particular strength of mine going all the way back to when I was in my mother's womb. No—this option would be too close to a date. There would be too much pressure.

*Heeelp! I don't know what to do!*

I ended up going inside Mr. Subb with Kristen. We ate there and had a lovely conversation. My worries had been much ado about nothing.

Now that the ice had a hairline crack, our lab interactions were less forced (forced on my part; Kristen could communicate like a well-adjusted adult). One chat started with an innocent question about weekend plans that somehow got all bent out of shape and became a date night in Lake George. What!? That was not part of the plan! I was ill-prepared for a formal date in a resort town that was an hour away! And besides, I wasn't collecting Social Security yet!

But the date was on. So the next day, I called my sister-in-law for advice on what I should wear. She steered me away from going with my trademark "uncoordinated casual" look, a fashionable and endearing outfit consisting of gym shorts and a concert T-shirt that rarely matched (I'm colorblind). We settled on jean shorts and a polo shirt, which I would have to purchase.

After buying the high-end attire, I moved on to the next item on my pre-date checklist: creating a mixtape for the drive to Lake George. This way, there would be less pressure to engage in conversation. The prospect of this date had me freaked out.

The date was very relaxing and enjoyable. We went to dinner, walked around Lake George, and listened to a Jimmy Buffet cover band at a lounge. Again, my worries were much ado about nothing.

The first date led to a second date, a third, a fourth . . . Nothing unusual— just two people getting to know each other and falling in love.

Now we'll fast-forward two and a half months from our first date to November 6, 1992. It was a typical Friday night, which meant that we sat on a couch in my apartment and assessed the state of our relationship. You didn't misread that. I have no idea why I initiated those conversations. We would talk about the present, the future, past relationships, past experiences, and what we were looking for in a relationship.

The conversation that evening was just like the others. Then it took a sharp turn. Here's what happened (in screenplay form):

FADE IN:

EXT. TWO-STORY APARTMENT BUILDING — 1992 — NIGHT

A peaceful night. The camera zooms in on a second-floor apartment window.

INT. APARTMENT, FAMILY ROOM — NIGHT

A dimly lit bachelor pad with hand-me-down furniture and a dartboard. MARK, 23, tall, socially awkward, sits on a couch next to his girlfriend KRISTEN, 22, beautiful brunette, not socially awkward. R.E.M. plays on the stereo.

> MARK
>
> I don't know. Hopefully, I'll land something soon and get my career started. I better 'cus my days working in the lumberyard are numbered. My contempt for wood products is beginning to reflect in my job performance.

> KRISTEN
>
> I'll miss seeing you in your dirty work boots.

> MARK
>
> That is my best look. How do you think things are going?

> KRISTEN
>
> With us?

                    MARK
Yeah. It's time for our weekly check-in.

Kristen smiles.

                  KRISTEN
I'm curious about our future. Were you
serious about moving to North Carolina?

                    MARK
Maybe. I'm not sure. It just seems like
a nice place to live. Great climate.
Something different than New York. Where
do you think you'll be in ten years?

                  KRISTEN
Married to you with six children.

Mark is stoic as he stares blankly ahead.

                                    CUT TO:

ANIMATION — MARK'S BRAIN AT WORK

A chaotic white web of brain synapses against a black
background. ONE MISSISSIPPI appears on the screen. Yellow
paths light up in the web as Mark's brain tries to establish a neural pathway that leads to a logical response
to the provocative stimulus it just received.

TWO MISSISSIPPI. Mark's brain is now a flurry of chaotic
neural activity as different pathways turn on and off.

THREE MISSISSIPPI. Bingo! A super-bright, yellow path cuts through the chaotic web as the other paths fade.

BACK TO:

INT. APARTMENT, FAMILY ROOM — NIGHT

Mark calmly looks at Kristen.

> MARK
>
> Do you want to get married?

Kristen is surprised as she studies his face.

> KRISTEN
>
> Seriously?

> MARK
>
> Yes.

> KRISTEN
>
> Okay.

> MARK
>
> Do you mean yes?

> KRISTEN
>
> Yes.

> MARK
>
> Are you sure?

<pre>
                    KRISTEN
      Yes, I'm sure. Are you sure?


                     MARK
      Yeah, I'm sure. Are you sure you're sure?
      I mean, I won't be offended if—


                    KRISTEN
      Mark, I love you!


                     MARK
      I love you too. Wow. So we're engaged.
</pre>

Kristen and Mark stare at each other in disbelief over what just transpired.

<pre>
                  END OF SCENE
</pre>

That's what happened on November 6, 1992. Two and a half months into our relationship, Kristen mentioned marriage in passing, and I felt compelled to propose for some mysterious reason.

I loved Kristen but had never thought about marriage before. Not a single thought. Why did I propose? I could have easily brushed off her comment about marrying and having six children. But I didn't. Why?

One year after we started dating, we were married. Over thirty years later, our relationship and love have never been stronger. It's perfectly imperfect.

Back to the central question: What possessed me to propose to Kristen on November 6, 1992? As I was writing this story, and reflecting on my marriage and what I had learned from this book, I finally solved the riddle!

When I proposed to Kristen, I wasn't *reacting* to what she had said about seeing herself married to me. Instead, my SAGe *responded* in a way that was true to my all-knowing spirit. This is what my SAGe knew that evening, even before my conscious mind had connected the dots:

○ I was madly in love with Kristen, and that love wouldn't fade over time, nor would her beauty.

○ Kristen was a deeply caring, kind, and loving person. She would be a wonderful wife and mother who always put family first.

○ Kristen would bring out my capacity to love selflessly. In many ways, loving selflessly has defined the most fulfilling aspect of my life. I didn't expect that.

○ Kristen and I would share the most important parts of our lives—raising our children, creating joyful moments with our family, making ends meet, and navigating all the stupid things life tosses your way. Everything in my life would be better with her than without her.

○ Kristen would support me as I pursued my dreams and overcame obstacles. And I would be there for her in kind.

○ Kristen would accept me and the perfection of all my imperfections. With Kristen, I could be authentic. And I would accept her in return.

○ Kristen and I would be compatible in mind and spirit. We shared the same values. We could be happy simply being around each other without saying a word.

○ Being with Kristen wouldn't always be frictionless. No relationship ever avoids conflict. Disconnects would occur, but love, communication, and compromise would remedy those.

On November 6, 1992, my Self-Actualized Genius knew I wanted to spend the rest of my life with Kristen.

○ ○ ○

# CHAPTER 14

# Are You Super-Connected?

## Relationships: What Are They Good For?
## Absolutely Everything!

Every living creature forms relationships with other creatures—within their species and across species—to sustain their lives. Just look at ants working together to create a thriving colony or a bee pollinating a flower. Relationships support basic needs like safety, nourishment, reproduction, and development.

Humans are a relationship-driven species. Throughout our evolutionary history, we have learned to flourish in social groups, relying on shared purpose and cooperation for survival. But the value of human relationships goes much deeper than that. Relationships provide one of the greatest opportunities for us to live the meaning of our lives, to feel and share love. Think about how you feel when you catch up with a good friend, help someone in need, or warmly embrace a loved one.

A relationship—whether it's between life partners, family, friends, acquaintances, coworkers, or even pets—represents the intersection of two lives.

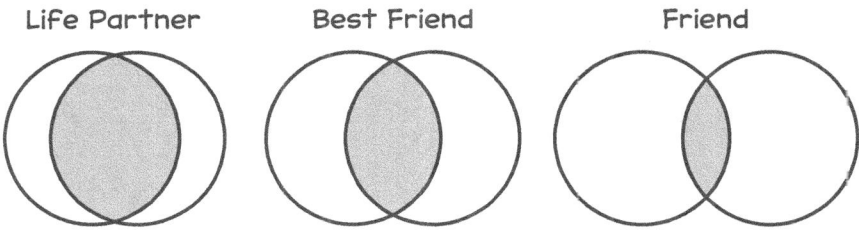

Life Partner    Best Friend    Friend

The overlapping sections in the Venn diagrams symbolize what two people share, including values, love, responsibilities, experiences, trust, and more. If you have a life partner, you'll want the overlap to be significant and represent your compatibility and love, which can keep your relationship satisfying for a lifetime.

But before we go further, I can tell you're jonesing for hard-core academic analysis to substantiate the value of relationships. So to keep our author-reader relationship healthy, I'll share some fascinating longitudinal research.

In the famous Harvard Study of Adult Development, a study that started in 1938 and tracked the lives of 724 Harvard students over their lifetimes—a study that is still active to this day—researchers found that the quality of social connections was the best predictor of a person's health and happiness throughout their life.

In a 2015 TED Talk, the study's director, Dr. Robert Waldinger, said, "The clearest message we get from this 75-year study is this: Good relationships keep us happier and healthier . . . It turns out that people who are more socially connected to family, to friends, to community are happier, they're physically healthier, and they live longer than people who are less well connected. And the experience of loneliness turns out to be toxic."[1]

If you scan the research or think about your own experience, you'll find overwhelming proof that healthy relationships add immense value to your life. I'll rattle off examples of that value: Relationships can boost your happiness and fulfillment. They create love. Relationships can make you feel secure, improve your health, reduce stress, help you live longer, and enrich your experiences. I could go on, but the evidence is staggering: **Healthy relationships are essential to nurturing the wonderful gift of your existence.**

Ready for a model? That was a silly question. Of course you are!

## The LAST Model in *The Wellness Ethic!*

Here's the LAST installment in your burgeoning collection of Wellness Ethic models:

# The LAST Relationship Model

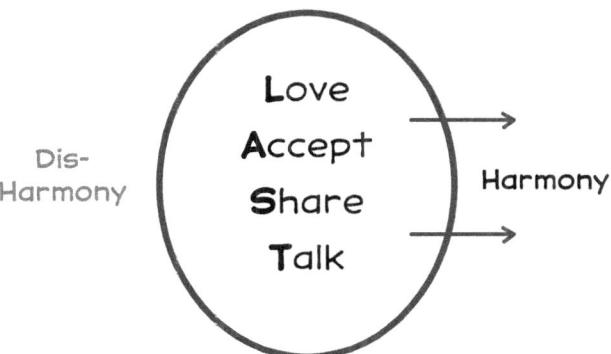

The LAST Relationship Model covers the fundamentals of a rewarding relationship that will LAST. Relationships thrive when two people foster *love* in their feelings and interactions, *accept* the perfection of their imperfections, *share* things in their lives in meaningful ways, and *talk* (communicate) to deepen their emotional connection and work through disharmony. That's the 80/20 of what it takes to maintain harmonious relationships.

The LAST Relationship Model applies to all types of relationships—the principles are universal—but the application can be scaled to reflect the importance of your connection. For example, if you have a life partner, love should be nurtured daily. With friends, love matters, and you'll want them to feel loved (or liked—however you want to describe your affection) through your words and actions. But you could go for weeks without speaking with most of your friends and not miss a beat. Let's unwrap the model.

# Harmony and Disharmony

In music, harmony is the blending of complementary tones that creates a sound pleasing to the human ear. In relationships, harmony is defined by how well two people's connection satisfies both parties. Take a few minutes and reflect upon the relationships that bring the most satisfaction to your life. What makes them tick?

The magic formula you came up with was probably in the ballpark of this: Your best relationships are marked by love, trust, and kindness. You share values. Your interests are compatible. You're both supportive. There's an ease and joy in your interactions. You accept and respect each other and can be authentic when together. You've found ways to work through friction without holding a grudge. We could add more to the list, but what I described gets to the heart of what makes relationships harmonious.

Now that you're feeling warm and gooey, we'll do a reality check: Life is imperfect, and since relationships are a part of life, relationships are imperfect. We know that mastering human interaction isn't easy. People are complex and have different values and personalities. They have different motivations, preferences, and interests. And here's the relationship kicker: Once you feel like you've figured out a lovely human being, they change on you. How dare they! You invested all that time adapting to their goofball behavior, and then they have the audacity to live life and grow. The question becomes: Will your relationship also grow to keep up with the changes in your lives?

Disharmony will creep into relationships. If the conflict is serious, and you let it fester, it could cause significant distress. Unresolved disharmony can also lead to the end of a relationship, which isn't always a bad outcome. Sometimes, phasing out a relationship is for the best, especially if it's toxic with little hope of recovery. But most times, your best option is to heal the fissure and restore harmony.

## **Love** – Accept – Share – Talk

Love is a passionate feeling of affinity that stirs the spirit. It defines the meaning of our lives. In a relationship, when you *feel love* for someone, your affection is characterized by a deep, emotional sense of connection, devotion, and care. You enjoy their company. You want the best for them. When they're happy, your day is lifted. When they suffer, you want to ease their suffering. Your love may extend to physical attraction if the person is a romantic interest.

When you *share your love* with others, you create special moments that generate loving experiences for them. It can be celebrating someone's birthday to show you care, being a comforting shoulder to cry on, or simply giving a sincere compliment. Your kind actions help others feel love in their lives, which, in turn, makes you feel even more love in your life.

> *Shared joy is a double joy; shared sorrow is half a sorrow.*
> —Swedish proverb

Thriving relationships are saturated in love. To nurture a loving relationship, we can apply what we learned in the "Love the Universe of Existence" section in chapter 8. If you love the universe of existence, you, by definition, love your relationships. In that section, we covered six concepts: *love yourself, appreciate your Mona Lisa moments, lead with love, practice radical gratitude, purge the dispiriting virus from your life,* and *feel connected to the universe of existence.* We'll explore each in the context of relationships.

As part of that exploration, I'll offer a counter-argument to Paul Simon's classic song "50 Ways to Leave Your Lover" by listing fifty ways that you can bring more love into your relationships. For the record, Mr. Simon only covered five ways to leave your lover in his song (*You just slip out the back, Jack . . .*). I'll beat his pedestrian total by forty-five! Just don't put my version to music. It's not hummable. I tried. For several months.

This is how I'll approach it. For each *love the universe of existence* concept, I'll offer an excerpt from chapter 8 that captures its essence, followed by a quick translation to show how the concept applies to relationships. Then, I'll list ways you could promote love. Miraculously, that will all need to add up to fifty. Remind me never to trash-talk the legendary Paul Simon again!

## Love Yourself

*Love starts and ends with you. In between is the love you share with others. When you love yourself, you embrace your spiritual essence as good. You know you have a lot to offer the world. You believe that you deserve happiness and fulfillment, and you move your life in a direction that realizes that promise.*

Relationship Translation: Promoting love in a relationship is challenging if you don't love yourself first. Start with self-love, then branch out from that position of loving strength.

1. Repeat daily affirmations that you are worthy of love.

2. Summon your SAGe and choose a positive frame and a self-loving response when you doubt or criticize yourself.

3. Celebrate wins in your life, no matter if they are big or small.

4. Embrace a healthy body image; accept the perfection of your creation.

5. Develop daily rituals that bring little doses of happiness into your life—drink delicious tea, take a warm bath, read uplifting books.

6. Create a lengthy list of your positive attributes. Ask others to share what they admire about you. Keep the list accessible, and go to it often.

7. Forgive yourself for past regrets. We have all made mistakes.

8. Spend time with people who love and encourage your authentic self.

9. Practice meditation and mindfulness to foster a sense of peace and love within your spirit.

10. Align your thoughts and actions with your values.

11. Find a way to move forward with your dreams, even if you take baby steps at first.

12. Refuse to compare yourself to others. No one has ever lived your unique life, so the comparison would be pointless.

13. Buy yourself a pet monkey—if you think that will bring you joy—but first confirm it's legal to own a primate in the jurisdiction in which you reside.

14. Say "no" to something to say "yes" to something more important.

15. Resurrect a childhood joy—playing a game you loved, drawing, collecting baseball cards—and be happy as you get lost in the activity.

16. Seek therapy, if necessary. Professional support can help you nurture self-love.

## Appreciate Your Mona Lisa Moments

*Each moment in your life can be a Mona Lisa moment if you appreciate what the universe offers you and mindfully engage your senses. Doing so helps you feel love in the present.*

Relationship Translation: In the moment, mindfully cherish the love, beauty, and joy that spring from your relationships.

17. Spend time with a loved one and mindfully engage in your interaction. Appreciate their voice and the love you share. Focus on the oneness you feel with them. What a gift they are to your life!

18. Appreciate your interactions with coworkers—their sense of humor, friendship, helpfulness, expertise, and your shared mission.

19. Go on a vacation with friends or family members. Create the conditions to experience many Mona Lisa moments.

20. Mindfully engage in your interactions with pets. Notice their gratitude when you feed them or how they respond when you give them loving attention. How does it make you feel?

## Lead with Love

*When you lead with love, you lead with empathy and care. You recognize that everyone has stuff going on in their life that you're not privy to. You realize that everyone is imperfect and deserves a break. You believe that everyone deserves love, including yourself. You choose a love-centered response to life that creates the best outcomes for everyone involved.*

Relationship Translation: Have love be your default position. Share your love often. Bring kindness, compassion, patience, and forgiveness to your relationships.

21. When you interact with a stranger, imagine they have a family, dreams, and a need to be loved. They're just like you. Interact kindly and notice their spirits lift. How does it make you feel?

22. Practice random acts of kindness regularly. Send a thoughtful gift or a kind handwritten note to a friend. Buy supplies for a teacher.

23. Use loving words in your conversations. Describe a person as amazing, awesome, beautiful, brilliant, caring, charming, considerate, creative, delightful, fascinating, funny, generous, humble, kind, lovely, patient, radiant, special, and other words that make them feel good.

24. Buy someone you love a pet monkey—if you think that will bring them joy—but first confirm it's legal to own a primate in the jurisdiction in which they reside.

25. Forgive someone who wronged you in your past. Help them move on with their life while learning from your loving example.

26. Be a servant leader at work. Understand the needs of those around you and make it your mission to serve them. Build your reputation for service, teamwork, helpfulness, and generosity.

27. Plan a special day for someone you love, including their favorite activities and foods. Leave no doubt that you love and appreciate them.

28. When someone is rude or insensitive to you, don't internalize their words. Choose a kind, uplifting response. Rise above the fray to bring peace to the relationship.

29. Recognize milestones and successes of others. Find ways to make people feel loved when something important happens in their lives.

30. Provide selfless support to someone who needs help—be an empathetic friend or lend a hand without being asked.

31. Share your good fortune with others. If you get a raise or bonus at work, give a portion to charity or take a friend to dinner.

## Practice Radical Gratitude

*A SAGe may want more in their life, whether it's finding more inner peace, having more financial security, or experiencing more adventure. But the SAGe is radically grateful for the blessings they already have and believes they don't really need anything else to be satisfied.*

Relationship Translation: Be thankful for the perfection of your imperfect relationships.

32. Reach out to someone you love and tell them why you love them.

33. Display pictures of your family, friends, and pets at home and work. Rotate the images to keep them fresh. Surround yourself with love.

34. Express your sincere gratitude every time someone helps you. Appreciate the good fortune of each loving interaction.

35. Create a gratitude journal and note what you're grateful for daily, including what's happening in your relationships.

## Purge the Dispiriting Virus from Your Life

*Wherever you're at, the dispiriting virus is constantly wrestling with your SAGe for control of you. The dispiriting virus wants you to live in the depths of despair. After all, misery loves company. When you love the universe of existence—when your life force is saturated with love—you choose better company, and your life takes off in wonderful and unexpected ways.*

Relationship Translation: Recognize when negativity from a relationship is overwhelming your spirit, and address the issue productively.

36. Accept that relationships will have negativity in them occasionally. Don't let it crush your spirit.

37. When a relationship has issues, take responsibility for your opportunities, apply your growth mindset, and learn from the experience.

38. If a relationship breaks down, utilize your emotional intelligence and partner with the other person to resolve the conflict.

39. Establish relationship boundaries when necessary.

40. Seek the support of a third party to mediate difficult issues with others.

41. When necessary, respectfully scale back or end a toxic relationship as an act of self-love.

42. If you made the ill-advised decision to buy a pet monkey (I was joking when I suggested it previously—I thought you knew that), and he's creating chaos in your life, try professional counseling to find common ground with the primate. If you're at an impasse and must part ways, negotiate a settlement to determine who keeps the house.

## Feel Connected to the Universe of Existence

*When you feel connected to the universe of existence, you recognize that you are an integral part of a greater whole. You love life, care for all living things, and strive to alleviate suffering. You understand that life isn't just about you; there's a bigger picture centered around creating harmony with humanity and nature to propagate love in the universe.*

Relationship Translation: The world provides unlimited opportunities to build loving and joyful relationships. But you must take the initiative.

43. Join clubs or social groups and do what you love to do with others.

44. Volunteer with a nonprofit and help others in need.

45. Mentor a child or a coworker.

46. Visit a nursing home and spend time with the elderly.

47. Walk around a park, a mall, or anywhere people are. Be an observer. Soak in humanity. Revel in the joy of others.

48. Pick up trash at a park, a beach, or a roadside to beautify nature and help wildlife thrive.

49. Mindfully engage with living things in nature. Embrace the wondrous diversity and symbiosis.

50. Hug a loved one—often—and connect with the comforting feeling.

I did it—that's fifty ways! Now I have a challenge for you: Begin a daily streak of bringing more love into your relationships. I provided a list of ideas to get you started, but be creative and expand upon it.

## Love – **Accept** – Share – Talk

After a few years of marriage, my family moved from New York to Ohio as part of a job relocation. My wife, Kristen, left her parents and siblings behind.

After the move, Kristen would travel to New York to visit her family. I usually didn't go with her, even though that wasn't her preference. I got along very well with my in-laws but cherished immersing myself in screenwriting when I had time off—making progress on my dreams was vital to my well-being. I was always grateful Kristen accepted that.

When you accept something, you acknowledge its existence without necessarily agreeing with what it represents. You may not even fully understand it. In a relationship, accepting a person means respecting them for who they are, including their differences with you and their perceived faults. When you accept a person and their behavior, you don't judge or try to change them.

**Acceptance is a choice.** When two people have a difference in values, priorities, opinions, behaviors, or personalities, both parties have a choice: Accept the difference and move on without letting it create friction, or don't accept the difference and deal with the fallout.

## Option 1: Accept the Difference

We're all unique people. My authentic, quirky self is different from your authentic, quirky self. I want you to respect me for who I am, and you deserve my respect as well.

So when you interact with me, expect to deal with a person who has a bone-dry sense of humor (which you may not always get, but then again, my humor confuses me as well), a horrible sense of direction (I will get us lost if you're foolish enough to ask me to navigate), a drive to go after my dreams (it impacts my availability to do things together), and an intense dislike for cheese (I need special consideration if I eat at your house). I told you I was quirky! Thankfully, the important people in my life accept me for who I am.

To lead yourself to acceptance of another person, you can:

○ *Embrace diversity.* The universe intentionally created diversity in abundance. Imagine a world with no diversity—sameness everywhere and in everything. That would be a dull world! Celebrate diversity.

○ *Treat others how you would like to be treated.* You would want people to give you space to be authentic, so return the favor.

○ *Have acceptance be your default position.* It is often the path of least resistance. Choose to accept unless you're given a good reason not to.

○ *View acceptance as a higher calling.* Summon your SAGe and all its wisdom to determine how to get to "yes" with acceptance.

○ *Keep perspective.* Is an issue or difference with someone worth becoming unhappy to the point that your dissatisfaction festers? Or is acceptance (or tolerance) the happy path?

○ *Choose kindness.* Will acceptance help the other person without harming you? If so, create love in the universe and accept.

Acceptance reflects emotional and spiritual strength. But sometimes acceptance would be too dissatisfying. That takes us to the next option:

## Option 2: Don't Accept the Difference

When you choose not to accept something, your next step is determining what to do about it. You can attempt to resolve the conflict or let the issue fester. We'll take the second option off the table since a SAGe wouldn't choose the unhappy path when there is a better alternative.

When you do not accept something, your objective should be to navigate the situation to get the best possible outcome. In some cases, such as being in a physically abusive relationship, it's critical to leverage the support of people who are trained to help.

But in most nonthreatening situations, the preferred path is to resolve the conflict by partnering with the other person to identify a solution that works for both parties. Examples include establishing a budget for a family member who struggles with overspending, agreeing to a reasonable curfew with a teenager who comes home late, or setting boundaries for a friend who borrows money but forgets to repay. We'll cover conflict resolution in the *talk* step of the LAST Relationship Model, so more on that soon.

If your attempts at conflict resolution fail, then the friction remains. Both parties then need to determine what that means to the relationship. If it's a serious matter, like a spouse unwilling to change their workaholic ways or address anger management issues, the disconnect could erode the relationship, possibly ending it, if progress isn't made. Or for less serious problems, should tolerance come into play, knowing that you don't have to agree on everything with someone to coexist peacefully? What would your SAGe advise?

When you task your love-centered SAGe to deal with relationship conflict, you'll be guided down a path that puts you in the best position for happiness.

## Love – Accept – **Share** – Talk

Your relationships are largely defined by what is shared. Here are some examples of things people share:

| | | |
|---|---|---|
| o Adventure | o Friends & Family | o Respect |
| o Altruism | o Hobbies & Interests | o Responsibilities |
| o Causes & Politics | o Lifestyle Choices | o Sacrifice |
| o Communication Style | o Love | o Secrets |
| o Culture | o Memories | o Sense of Humor |
| o Dreams & Objectives | o Money Matters | o Suffering |
| o Emotional Intimacy | o Personality | o Trust & Loyalty |
| o Experiences | o Physical Intimacy | o Values |
| o Faith & Spirituality | o Professional Pursuits | |

The best relationships are between two people whose expectations of each other are met. They are compatible in the areas that matter to them. That doesn't mean they are carbon copies of each other. They could have different personalities, politics, spiritual beliefs, you name it. But through it all, they've figured out how to share the intersection of their lives in a satisfying way that creates love and harmony and minimizes discord.

One way people share in a relationship is by *engaging in everyday interactions*. These are the ongoing connections that keep a relationship vibrant and fulfilling. They include conversations, experiences, and the simple joy of spending time together.

Another way to share is by *providing support*—emotionally and through words and actions—to help another person have the best possible outcome with whatever is going on in their life. When you support someone, you often feel love when you help them, but that's a side benefit. Your primary objective is to selflessly support the person for their benefit. That support could be in the form of helping someone through a difficult breakup, motivating a person to stay on track with exercising, providing financial assistance, or the much-dreaded offering a hand to move furniture.

When you provide support, you're sharing *you*—your love, time, talents, encouragement, resources, and wisdom. That's powerful. It's exciting. Your support has a meaningful impact on a person's life, sometimes a transformational one. It helps people feel like they matter and that they're loved. Providing support strengthens the ties that bind a relationship.

A third way to share in a relationship is by *partnering on a common mission*. When people engage at that level, they are mutually invested in the mission, and their emotional connection increases. Think about how you feel toward classmates who shared the coming-of-age experience with you, a life partner who has been lovingly by your side throughout life's successes and sorrows, or a work colleague who was in the trenches with you on a big project.

When two people row in the same direction on a common mission, it sets the stage for a deeper relationship. They share the journey of the partnership, both the triumphs and setbacks. Their mutual dependence strengthens their belief that they're "in it together." Shared memories are created. Trust and love grow in the fertile ground.

To nurture healthy relationships, consider what is shared. How are you connecting in your everyday interactions? Are you getting the support you need from others? Have you asked your family, friends, or work colleagues what support they need from you? How about the missions in your life that you partner with others to fulfill? Are those partnerships thriving? What can be done to bring more satisfaction into your partnerships? Every step forward that you take in your relationships improves your life and the lives of others.

A healthy relationship is balanced and loving. Each person has accepted what they can and has worked through what they cannot in a way that minimizes friction. They have kind and respectful interactions. Both parties feel like they're supported with what matters, and they partner on the important stuff in a satisfying way. Those are relationship conditions that help love flourish.

But as we know, everything can be rosy, and then disruption enters the room, bumps into the table, and topples our carefully constructed house of cards. People change. Relationships change. We lose focus. Stupid things happen. Issues appear. Dissatisfaction takes root. That brings us to communication and its indispensable role in maintaining the health of a relationship.

## Love – Accept – Share – **Talk**

Effective communication (*talk*)—verbal and nonverbal—is essential to a harmonious relationship. If love can be considered a relationship's life partner, communication can be regarded as its best friend. Communication conveys what is on a person's mind and how they feel. It reveals the authentic person. When done well, love and connection with another person are nurtured. When it breaks down, it can set a relationship back or even be its death knell.

There are many reasons why we communicate, including:

○ *Communicate to share love.* What is communicated and how it's conveyed creates an emotional feeling. Will affection and care define that feeling? Will both parties feel emotionally validated?

○ *Communicate to connect on a personal level.* Every person is interesting. They've had blessings and misfortunes. What makes them happy? What are they struggling with? What are they pursuing? When people connect personally, they show a genuine interest in each other. They find connections that help them relate. They build trust and affection.

○ *Communicate to work together and promote alignment.* When two people convey their needs, perspectives, and boundaries, they lay the foundation for a productive relationship. When they embrace compromise and maintain an open and collaborative dialogue, they promote a win-win partnership.

○ *Communicate to work through friction.* When a relationship is defined by healthy communication, issues are addressed when they're smaller. They tend not to fester. When a problem surfaces, both parties are accustomed to working through disconnects to recapture harmony.

Though most of us are well intentioned when communicating, we don't always get it right. We sometimes choose the wrong words or tone. We misread the needs of our audience. Our body language confuses. Or our Mischief Mind asserts itself, allowing our charged emotions to reduce our communication ability to the level of a grunting Neanderthal. And all that stuff is just on our end. Everything I listed could also be going on with the other person!

So many variables are at play that it would be unreasonable to expect people to communicate flawlessly. That's why grace, patience, and tolerance are admirable qualities when relating with others. We're all trying to connect as best we can in our imperfect way. But that doesn't absolve us from our responsibility to communicate well. That's what we'll cover now.

In staying true to the 80/20 rule, I'll focus on five essential communication topics that help maintain harmony in a relationship: (1) *communication styles*, (2) *confirmation bias*, (3) *negative interactions*, (4) *effective communication practices*, and (5) *conflict resolution*. You won't become a master communicator by reading this section, but you should pick up insights that will help you artfully use communication to strengthen your relationships.

## Communication Styles

A person's communication style influences the way they relate with people. By understanding your style and the style of others, you can tailor your interactions to navigate communication pitfalls while fostering empathy and connection. There are four primary communication styles:

○ *Passive:* Passive communicators don't freely offer opinions or share feelings. When communicating with a passive person, patiently ask questions to build trust and encourage them to engage.

○ *Aggressive:* Aggressive communicators tend to be domineering, reactionary, and direct. When relating with an aggressive communicator, set a positive tone from the onset to defuse potential aggression Then, use your emotional intelligence to assert your perspective and needs while managing the conversation's emotional charge.

○ *Passive-aggressive:* Passive-aggressive people are prone to hiding their true motives. Their words may not always align with their intent or actions. When communicating with a passive-aggressive person, clarify your understanding of what they say and root out unstated feelings, needs, and intentions.

○ *Assertive:* Assertive communicators relate by being open with their feelings and needs while respecting others. Be clear, direct, and respectful when engaging with an assertive person.

We'll look at an example: Laticia works long hours as a banking executive and is behind on a major project. Her tenth-grade son fought at school, so she must attend a meeting with his principal. Laticia's husband is joining her. When Laticia is stressed, she can be aggressive. Do you think that tendency could negatively impact her interactions at the meeting? You bet.

But it's not a lost cause. If Laticia were self-aware of her habit of being aggressive in stressful situations, she could moderate her communication style to create a better outcome. If the principal, husband, and son were also aware of her challenges, they could intentionally set a positive tone from the onset. They could then counter her aggressiveness by using their emotional intelligence to manage the conversation's emotional charge as they assert their perspective. By doing so, they would help shape a productive interaction.

## Confirmation Bias

Confirmation bias occurs when people seek out and interpret information in a manner that validates their preexisting beliefs while discounting information that runs counter to those beliefs. Human brains don't like to be wrong and can distort reality to avoid such unpleasantness.

For instance, if you think I'm a slob, you'll probably notice my slob-like behavior, even if my infractions are infrequent. And you'll discount the times I vacuum the house, do the dishes, care for the yard, and keep my home office immaculate because those examples contradict your entrenched belief. (Are you reading this, Kristen? I have made strides!)

To overcome confirmation bias, shun broad generalities, explore diverse perspectives, and engage in critical thinking. Look for factual evidence as you open your mind and seek the unbiased truth.

## Negative Interactions

In his book *The Seven Principles for Making Marriage Work*, Dr. John M. Gottman identified four types of negative interactions between a couple: criticism, contempt, defensiveness, and stonewalling.[2] All four have the potential to stifle the love between two people if left unaddressed. Here's a breakdown:

- ○ *Criticism:* Criticism is the act of passing judgment, often by revealing perceived shortcomings in an action or behavior. It can be delivered constructively and compassionately, inspiring a spirit of cooperation in addressing the issue, or it can be communicated in a judgmental and demoralizing manner, creating a negative interaction.

  Examples (delivered poorly): *You always screw things up. You should have known better. I can't rely on you. You clearly don't care. If I want something done right, I have to do it myself.*

- ○ *Contempt:* When a person feels contempt toward someone, they often show disgust and disrespect or act with an air of superiority. You may see eye-rolling or hear sarcasm and belittling comments. Contempt usually signifies a deeper issue in a relationship.

  Examples: *You'll never amount to anything. You're so dumb. You disgust me. You're incompetent. I wish I had never met you.*

- ○ *Defensiveness:* People who act defensively fail to take accountability for their actions. They tend to blame others, deny responsibility, and make excuses. The root cause of this behavior can be low self-esteem, insecurity, or the fear of being wrong or rejected. It can also result from how a person was spoken to during a conversation (harsh language can immediately put someone in a defensive posture).

  Examples: *I didn't do anything wrong; you screwed it up. I tried my best; you're just being critical. Why do you always judge me? No one helped me—what did you expect? You're too sensitive.*

○ *Stonewalling*: When someone stonewalls during a conflict, they withdraw or shut down. Telltale signs of stonewalling include avoiding eye contact, being silent, giving short answers to questions, showing indifference, or disengaging completely. Stonewalling prevents issues from being addressed and undermines emotional connection.

Examples (if anything is even said): *I won't discuss this further. I don't have to explain myself to you. I don't care.*

When negative interactions occur, it is important that both parties engage in an open and respectful dialogue to understand the behavior, its root causes, and the impact on the relationship. Being vulnerable and sharing feelings during the discussion can lead to a breakthrough. To bring emotions to the forefront, use phrasing like: *"When you do [negative behavior], I feel [specific emotion]."* That makes the negative behavior more personal. It shows that a real person is negatively impacted. It underscores the need for change.

Once the truth is understood, the focus can then turn to improving interactions moving forward. The rest of this chapter will help with that.

## Effective Communication

There are many aspects of effective communication; I'll offer six potent ones:

○ *Practice active listening.* When you actively listen, you seek to understand what the other person says. You get insights that inform your perspective and help shape your response. You build trust and respect. Here are some tenets of active listening:

• Pay attention to what is being said without focusing on your response.

- Avoid interruptions that break a train of thought.

- Don't pass judgment.

- Provide verbal and nonverbal cues that you're listening.

- Ask questions to probe deeper.

- Recap key points to confirm understanding.

○ *Be respectful, empathetic, and kind in your interactions.* By taking a positive approach, you're letting the other person know that you respect and care for them and that you'll play your part in resolving friction when it occurs. Positivity is a catalyst for cooperation.

○ *Guide the conversation with emotional intelligence.* An emotionally intelligent person is aware of the emotional charge of a discussion and guides emotions within themselves and others to a productive place.

○ *Be open and honest.* The more open and honest both parties are in a conversation, the more productive it will be. Without candor, the substance of a conversation will be disguised or misunderstood.

○ *Pay attention to the nonverbals.* When people communicate, nonverbal cues—avoiding eye contact, rolling eyes, smiling, nodding in agreement, looking at a cell phone, seething—can speak louder than what is said. Ensure your nonverbal cues convey what you intend. If you pick up on a nonverbal cue from someone that is concerning, address it in a nonaccusatory manner to see if your perception was correct, and then work on the root cause if necessary.

○ *Confirm agreements and next steps.* After a substantive conversation, confirm what was decided and how you'll move forward. A clear confirmation that expresses genuine optimism increases the odds that both parties will stay aligned.

## Conflict Resolution

Conflict can occur in every aspect of your personal and professional life. Conflict resolution skills are a coveted superpower—some people make careers out of their ability to get people on the same page. It's also a competency that can be learned. I'll share a conflict resolution process that can help you take a partnering approach to resolving issues:

*Step 1: Set a productive tone for partnering.* Choose a proper setting with a good ambience. Start the discussion with positive sentiments, like expressing that you value the relationship and are confident that the issue will be resolved. Agree upon guiding principles to resolve the conflict, such as striving for a win-win solution, being respectful, listening without judgment, having an open mind, avoiding defensiveness, and keeping a big-picture perspective.

*Step 2: Seek to understand.* Have a productive conversation to deepen each person's understanding of the issue, its root cause, and its practical and emotional impact. Be empathetic, emotionally intelligent, and respectful throughout the discussion. Actively listen. Look for common ground; work through disconnects. Build trust as you both move closer in mind and spirit.

*Step 3: Ensure there's a shared will to resolve the issue.* If there's a shared will, there's a way, so proceed to the next step if that's the case. If not, then seek to understand why (5 Whys). Can the resistance be overcome? Could a third party help to get both parties on the same page (see Step 5)? If a shared will is not attainable, then further attempts to resolve the conflict may be futile until the root cause of the resistance is understood and addressed.

*Step 4: Explore solutions to the conflict and reach an agreement on a win-win resolution.* As options are explored, riff off each idea and see if a win-win resolution emerges. If a solution favors one party over the other, and the sacrifice from one person is too much to bear, can something be done creatively to make it work? Once a resolution meets the needs of both parties, confirm acceptance.

*Step 5: Involve a third party, if necessary.* If one of the parties doesn't have the will to work together or acceptable progress on a resolution is not being made, consider involving a third party, whether it's a counselor, a trusted friend, or a leader at work. Introducing a neutral party into the mix, especially a person skilled at resolving conflict, can often break through the gridlock.

*Step 6: Follow up and follow through to ensure sustained satisfaction.* As both parties move forward with the resolution, periodically check in to gauge if it's still working. Adjustments may need to be made as life happens, but that's normal—maintaining harmony requires ongoing care.

## Assessing Relationship Health

A healthy relationship has alignment between expectations and reality, and when there is a disconnect, the parties partner to find a satisfying path forward.

A helpful way to get your arms around the health of a relationship is to break it down in terms of the LAST Relationship Model—love, accept, share, and talk. What's working well when you look at a relationship from those perspectives? Is anything falling short of expectations? And what can be done to close important gaps?

We'll go through an example. Consider the fictitious but adorable married couple Mary and Leopold. Sadly, they have been drifting apart. An astute friend recommended they read *The Wellness Ethic* to see if it could help them get back on track. They read it (their five-star Amazon review characterized it as "a thick book that offers various insights on stuff") and were inspired to assess their relationship in terms of the LAST Relationship Model. To my delight, they tossed their thoughts into a nifty chart (I want to adopt this couple!):

| Love | Accept |
|---|---|
| - We have twenty years of a loving relationship.<br>- Our emotional connection has diminished over the past couple of years due to not spending enough quality time together. | - Mary accepts Leopold's role in their community's homeowners' association.<br>- Leopold doesn't accept Mary's long hours at work.<br>- Mary doesn't accept Leopold's passive-aggressive communication style.<br>- We do not accept that we don't spend enough time together. |
| **Share** | **Talk** |
| - We share parenting two teenagers, values and trust, household chores, passion for adventure, and binge-watching British crime dramas.<br>- Mary supports Leopold's lifestyle changes (diet and exercise).<br>- Leopold supports Mary's care of her elderly parents. | - Due to our busy schedules, we do not have casual conversations like we used to. We miss that.<br>- We are usually good at resolving conflict, but issues have festered lately.<br>- Leopold can be passive-aggressive.<br>- Mary has an assertive communication style. |

When they took stock of their chart, Mary and Leopold zeroed in on the *Love* and *Share* quadrants. They acknowledged that they had a strong foundation of love represented there. This put their problems in perspective—the issues were serious, but in the grand scheme, their challenges represented a fraction of their overall relationship. A lot was going well, and they were committed to making things better.

As they discussed their marriage against the backdrop of the chart, they identified two prime improvement opportunities: how they spend their time and Leopold's passive-aggressive communication style.

*How they spend their time.* They recognized they were overcommitted. As a result, they didn't spend much quality time together, which made them feel less connected to each other. Being overcommitted was also the root cause of their issues festering. The solutions: To free up time, Leopold resigned from his role in the homeowners' association, and Mary agreed to set more boundaries at work—if she couldn't strike a better work-life balance in the next six months, she would look for another job. They also scheduled a family vacation to Yellowstone to add adventure to their lives and agreed to take evening walks together to connect and decompress.

*Leopold's passive-aggressive communication style.* Mary provided examples to Leopold and then explained that it made her feel belittled, especially when he was condescending. Leopold was unaware that he had this tendency. The solutions: Leopold committed to improving. Mary asked permission to point out examples in the future if he ever backtracked. Leopold was on board with that and promised not to be defensive.

On top of implementing their solutions, Leopold and Mary agreed to discuss future issues in real time so they could proactively address them. They also decided to check in once a month to see how things were going in their marriage. They scheduled that during the time they reviewed their financial budget (habit stacking).

Mary and Leopold's tale showed that a healthy relationship requires nurturing. When issues crop up, both parties should keep love at the fore-front as they partner to get the relationship to a better place. If there's a shared will, there's a way.

○ ○ ○

## Move Forward on Your Wellness Ethic Journey!

① Assess the health of an important relationship in your life by filling out the LAST Relationship Assessment (include your counterpart in the exercise).

| Love | Accept |
|------|--------|
| Share | Talk |

② Detail what actions you'll both take to bring more harmony into your relationship (include change adoption approaches as appropriate).

③ Advanced Topics (going beyond the 80/20): Research the topics of "emotional intimacy" and "physical intimacy" to explore how the application of those concepts can help your relationships thrive.

## Mark's Example

(1) Assess the health of an important relationship in your life by filling out the LAST Relationship Assessment (include your counterpart in the exercise).

*Kristen + Mark's Relationship*

| Love | Accept |
|---|---|
| - Thirty years of a loving relationship built on care, affection, acceptance, partnership, support, trust, and fun. | - Kristen doesn't accept Mark's messiness.<br>- Mark doesn't accept Kristen's issues with managing money. |
| **Share** | **Talk** |
| - We share parenting, cats, values and trust, a quiet lifestyle and temperament, a passion for equality, and life experiences.<br>- Kristen supports Mark's side hustles and job demands.<br>- Mark supports Kristen's choice to be a stay-at-home mom and her pottery hobby. | - Our communications are positive and kind, emotionally intelligent, and issues are resolved in a timely manner.<br>- Both Kristen and Mark have assertive communication styles. |

(2) Detail what actions you'll both take to bring more harmony into your relationship (include change adoption approaches as appropriate).

> Work on areas we do not accept: Mark's messiness and Kristen's money management. We both take it seriously and are getting better, so it's a very minor annoyance in the big picture. We'll continue to give each other feedback and keep working it.

# Personal & Professional Pursuits

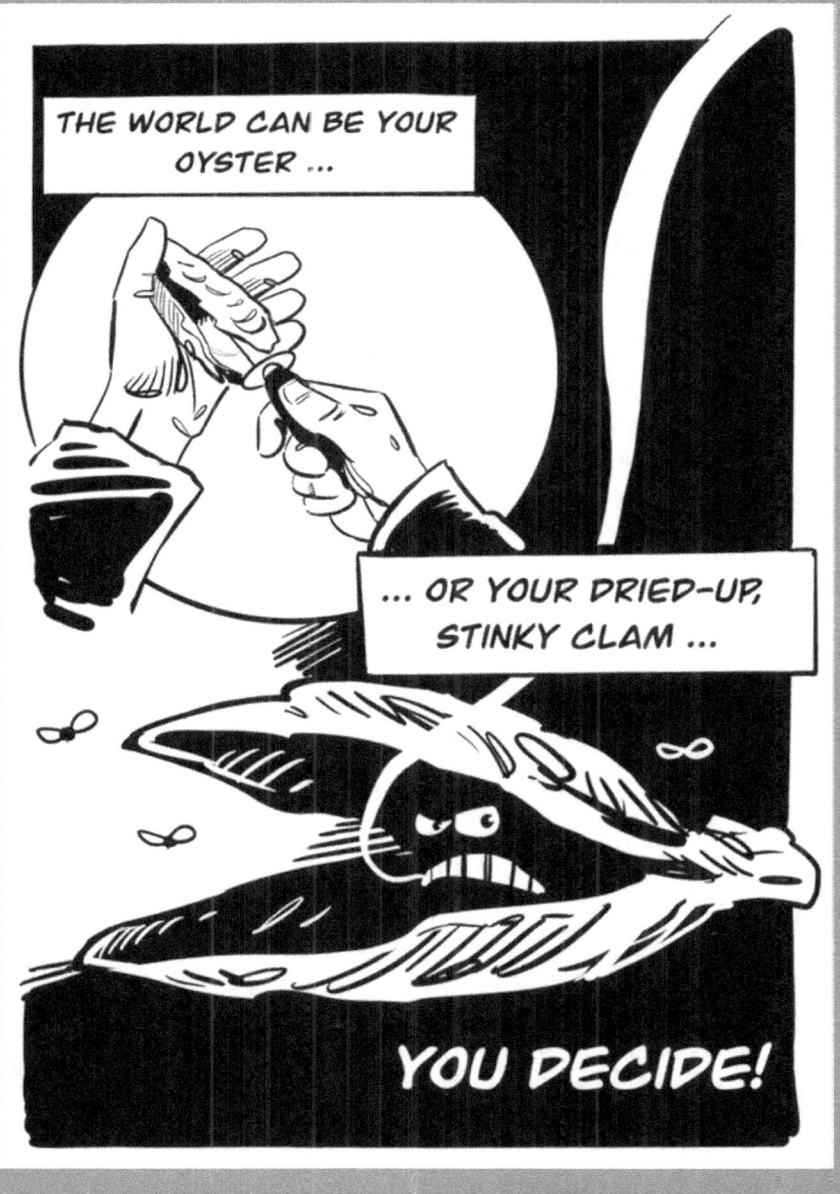

# CHAPTER 15

# A Story of Vision

Have you ever had a brilliant idea you were convinced would make you millions, maybe even billions? Assuming, of course, that you were bold enough to go after it. But at the time of idea conception, you're thinking: *Execution, schmexecution—don't bore me with those buzz-killing details!*

You envision your idea coming to fruition and your life being transformed. Your mind floats to la-la land as you imagine the riches that will surely come your way. You think about providing a comfortable life for your family and supporting nonprofits. You fantasize about having the freedom of time and money to pursue your dreams, preferably while living in a beautiful house on Lake Champlain with the serene Green Mountains looming in the distance.

I love to dream.

I've had dozens of money-making ideas over the decades that I thought were winners. I'll tell you about one that had enormous potential: Think *international buffet.* Okay, before you get all judgy on me and dismiss my once-in-a-generation restaurant concept, hear me out. The buffet would offer an international cuisine rotation—perhaps Monday would feature German, Thai, Peruvian, Spanish, and Irish; Tuesday would include British, Mongolian, Brazilian, Hungarian, and Ethiopian . . . On every visit, you could delight in diverse, delectable dishes from around the globe. There's something to my idea.

But I'm not gifted in culinary matters, except for the mad cooking skills I developed at Little Caesars Pizza and Taco Bell during high school. I never managed a restaurant beyond running a day shift. I also don't have millions of dollars sitting around twiddling their green ink-stained thumbs, waiting to fund a business venture. There was always a long procession of well-reasoned excuses not to open an international buffet, so I didn't. I'll always wonder: *What if I had?* I could have become the world-renowned Sultan of the Smorgasbord!

I hate what-ifs that become never-dids.

I had another business idea that I loved, which came to me in 2012. It started to germinate when I decided to invigorate my stale CD collection by going on Facebook and posting a request to my friends for music recommendations. My post drifted away in Facebook's sea of blah and generated few responses. What I really wanted to do was scroll through album reviews and top 10 lists from people I trusted, but content like that didn't exist.

I knew there had to be a better way to do social media. Then, I had a eureka moment while taking a shower (I know it's clichéd to come up with an idea while taking a shower, but I like to be clean, and sometimes novel thoughts enter my brain as I accomplish that worthy objective). The idea was to create a one-stop, network-based social media app that allowed members to post and browse reviews, top 10 lists, things for sale, and want ads. If content like that came from your network, it would be far more engaging and trustworthy than anything on Facebook (Facebook didn't offer features like that back then).

I had to explore the concept further, so I created a pitch that included wireframes (visual prototypes of the app), functional requirements, and a business case. I chose the name *Listersection* (the intersection of lists) for the app—I'd improve the name later. Here is one of the original wireframes:

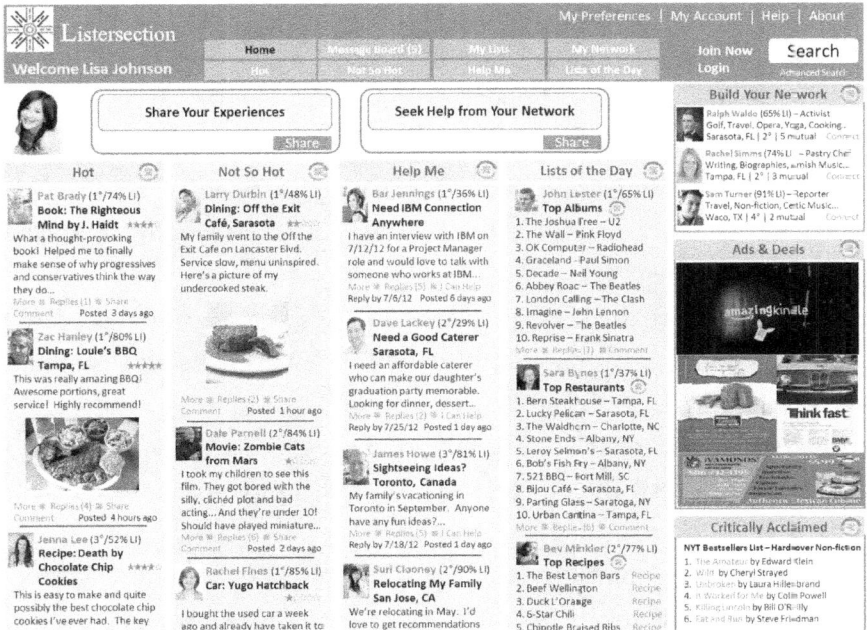

I didn't know what to do next. I had a start-up idea that I loved. The barriers to entry with launching a social media app were relatively low. But—get ready for a cavalcade of excuses—I didn't have money to invest. I didn't have free time to develop the idea. Facebook was a monopoly whose preference was not to be toppled. And I had no experience writing code or building an app.

The excuses won the argument. It looked like Listersection would meet the fate of my international buffet dream—a promising idea best executed by someone with courage and resourcefulness. After a few months, I confronted my fear of rejection and sent the pitch to a handful of business colleagues to see if one of them wanted to partner on it. I struck out. So I returned to my comfort zone: working at my day job and writing screenplays on weekends.

Listersection languished in the land of misfit start-up ventures for over a year. Then, on a whim, I sent an email with the Listersection pitch to a tech executive I had previously worked with—perhaps he could lead the technical build? This was a last-ditch effort to drum up interest. If he passed, the life support cord would be yanked, and my dream of squashing Facebook would end. To my utter shock, he replied that he was intrigued by the idea and wanted to discuss it further. What?! Holy cow! I had no idea if his curiosity would lead to anything, but at least my dream finally got a gulp of oxygen!

We met and chatted about the concept. He saw the business potential and wanted in as a co-founder. Without hesitation, I offered a fifty/fifty ownership split. Even though I had conceived of the idea and had a fairly mature vision, I knew the heaviest lift would be the tech build. I wanted to respect that. A fifty/fifty partnership would also serve as a motivator for him to be all-in.

We had more meetings to discuss the product roadmap and our role clarity. We agreed he would lead everything related to technology—coding, architecture, and infrastructure—as the Chief Technology Officer (CTO). I would serve as the Chief Product Officer and lead the product design and strategy. To create the space to go after this, I knew I couldn't afford to quit my corporate job. But I could put screenwriting on the back burner. The start-up was too thrilling to pass up, and something had to give. So one side hustle was put on hold to launch another.

Our bootstrapped start-up was operational from early 2014 through late 2017. I'll provide a summary view of the experience. To respect privacy, I'll leave names out. Everyone involved with the enterprise undoubtedly has a unique perspective on how it went. Here's how I saw it . . .

To give context, I'll share a sample screenshot from the desktop app we built (there was also a mobile web version). As you'll see, we landed on the name *Paloozoo*, a derivative of "palooza," which suggested that our site would have fun and diverse content. Note: Some of the names in the posts have been grayed out to protect privacy, and the Pet Boobah [*sic*] price is firm.

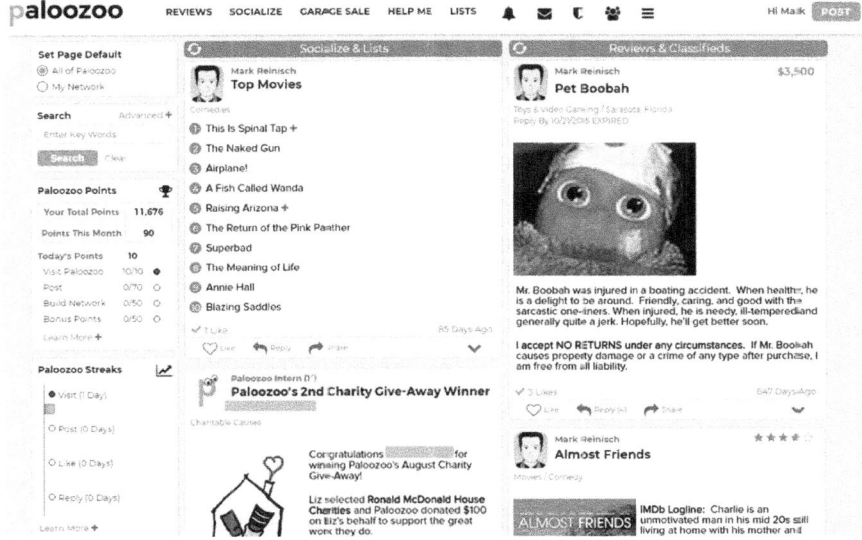

After launching Paloozoo, we thought it would take six to nine months to build a minimum viable product to release to the marketplace. The intent was to create a product with *just enough* features and functionality that a user would get sufficient value to want to return to the app. We would then build and roll out new features as we simultaneously marketed the app to attract more users. That approach looked great on paper. We were terribly naive.

We grossly underestimated how difficult it would be to extract users from Facebook—people already had fully formed networks there, and Facebook's app was feature-rich. Or how challenging it would be to motivate folks to add Paloozoo to their daily rotation of apps—our value proposition would have to resonate with them emotionally before they would go that far.

We also underestimated the effort required to build Paloozoo and run its operations. To give a better sense of the magnitude of the undertaking, the following is a list of software and business development activities we worked on. This list excludes many architecture and infrastructure efforts the CTO led—I trusted his considerable expertise on those matters.

## Software Development

o Sign Up & Account Administration
o Network Build & Manage Groups
o Products: Reviews, Socialize, Lists, Garage Sale & Help Me
o UX Design
o Saved Posts, Like, Reply & Share
o Gamification
o Content Search & Controls
o Paloozoo InMail & Notifications
o Facebook API

## Business Development

o LLC & Operating Agreement
o Board of Directors
o Patents & Trademarks
o Press Releases, Facebook Ads & Charity Contest
o Training & Marketing Videos
o Email Marketing
o Paloozoo Blog
o Privacy Policy
o Financial Management

When I look at that list, I'm amazed by how much effort we put into our start-up. Every software capability we built went through an exhaustive process of developing a concept, building out functional requirements, designing the user interface, coding (to make it functional), iterating on the design, testing, fixing bugs, and launching into production.

What added to the challenge was that most of the business and software development activities were new to me. So for the four years that Paloozoo existed, I committed around twenty hours a week to the venture, learned at a breakneck speed, and constantly expanded my capabilities. It was one of the most invigorating experiences of my life.

But the Paloozoo start-up was also one of the most frustrating experiences of my life. That was due to the people part, which was ultimately our undoing. Every deliverable required the CTO and me to get on the same page. We had equal decision-making authority but different visions and mindsets. It resulted in a contentious relationship, especially toward the end.

Our struggle to get new users to return after their first visit added to our frustration. When we marketed the site, we would get an uptick in sign-ups but rarely the coveted return visitor. So we would add new features, simplify the user experience, iterate on the design, add gamification, and try other approaches to grow our active user base. But those efforts were to limited avail.

After close to four years of development, Paloozoo was at a crossroads: If we couldn't solve our active user issue, we would need to consider shutting down the venture. I viewed Paloozoo's traction challenges as product-driven—the app had to be stickier. To accomplish that, we needed to provide a user experience that inspired users to return, which required making the app easier to use and more feature-rich. I also advocated gearing our app toward positive social media to differentiate it from the toxic social media that was prevalent at the time. Those pivots would require significant tech development.

The CTO disagreed with my direction and saw our issue as a marketing challenge: We needed to reach more users and get them to sign up. From my perspective, it didn't matter how many users signed up if they didn't use the app and return. We were at an impasse.

Our relationship had become too combative to work through our issues constructively, so we decided to shut down Paloozoo in the fall of 2017. Giving up on a dream was spiritually draining for me, especially after four years of devotion and sacrifice, but I carefully considered all options and felt it was best to move on.

After we stopped our development and marketing efforts, we worked with one of our board members and made a last-gasp attempt to get a financial return from our start-up. The board member contacted his network to see if anyone wanted to buy us out. I didn't expect anything to come of it. To my surprise, he found an interested buyer, an emergent entertainment company. They envisioned transforming Paloozoo into a social media app and movie streaming service for the independent film community.

After a month-long negotiation and due diligence process, we closed the deal in December 2017. Unbelievable! It was such an unexpected and gratifying outcome. As I wrote in the introduction to this book:

*Life is unpredictable. It's a potpourri of triumphs and struggles, with good fortune that bounces your way as if guided by Divinity, and stupid things thrown in your path by Chance.*

Many lessons were learned as I look back at the Paloozoo experience and put it through the Wellness Ethic lens. I'll share a few:

*One pursuit in your life rarely provides all the satisfaction you need, but you'll want the totality of your pursuits to fully satisfy you.* In my case, my corporate career was only a piece of my satisfaction puzzle. I needed more of a creative outlet than it provided, and I wanted autonomy to make a broader impact on the world. So I pursued side hustles to close the gaps. That approach wouldn't work for everyone, but it was what I needed to do to fulfill the vision I had for my life.

*You should tackle big challenges one step at a time.* The magnitude of what it took to build Paloozoo was intimidating. But by taking it step by step, we would reach a milestone. When we reached a few milestones, we would achieve an objective. String a couple of objectives together, and you've got serious momentum—step by step by step by step.

*You and I have unlimited capabilities.* I became the founder of a social media start-up. I did that despite having limited entrepreneurial experience. I couldn't code. I didn't have a product management background. I had a demanding corporate job. I had minimal funds. And I didn't even like social media! I kicked excuses to the curb to move forward with my vision. If an imperfect, challenged guy like me could find a way to launch Paloozoo—in partnership with a supremely talented team—**I'm confident you can accomplish practically anything you set your mind to.**

*A growth mindset and the ability to pivot are essential for life satisfaction (and start-up success).* Reality rarely unfolds as you had scripted. Your ability to accept that, learn from it, and adjust accordingly will impact your success in whatever you pursue.

*Relationships matter.* The Paloozoo start-up wouldn't have accomplished anything without the team we assembled. I am very grateful for the significant contributions of the CTO, VP of Operations, board members, experts, friends, and family. But we would have accomplished exponentially more had the CTO and I rowed in the same direction on strategy and found a way to expand our team to close skill and capacity gaps. Paloozoo was more about the people than it was about tech and innovation. I wish I had understood that at the time.

*Always prioritize your wellness, no matter what is going on in your life.* Pursuing Paloozoo as a side hustle was mentally, physically, and spiritually exhausting. But I can't imagine what it would have been like without exercising regularly, eating well, prioritizing sleep, sharing the Paloozoo journey with my family by involving them in the venture, and finding ways to de-stress. Wellness should never take a back seat to anything in your life.

With Paloozoo, I followed Thoreau's wise counsel and advanced confidently in the direction of my dreams for four years. I had hoped to capture a percentage or two of Facebook's market share and retire as a filthy rich billionaire—that seemed perfectly reasonable to me—but it didn't happen. However, failure isn't how I define our story now that I have put it through the Wellness Ethic lens. We met with a "success unexpected in common hours."

This is how I define my Paloozoo success: It was a gift to have the experience of being the founder of a tech start-up. It was fulfilling to go all-in on a dream with everything I had and grow my capabilities. It was thrilling to partner with a committed team and realize a crazy vision. Even the obstacles, sacrifices, and frustrations were important to my satisfaction because they added to the depth of the experience. The fact that we sold the business was a welcome bonus but not required for Paloozoo to be considered a success.

My stint as an entrepreneur also opened doors of opportunity. Paloozoo helped me land a desirable corporate job (it was all the CEO wanted to discuss during my interview), and it gave me the confidence and inspiration to tackle my next ambitious side hustle—this book!

All of that wasn't the success I had envisioned when I launched Paloozoo, but I'm happy with it. It was an opportunity to nurture the wonderful gift of my existence, and that's what I aspire to do with my life—that I control.

o   o   o

# CHAPTER 16

# It's All Personal . . . and It Can Be Professional Too

In William Shakespeare's seventeenth-century play *The Merry Wives of Windsor*, the knight Falstaff tells his crony, Pistol: "I will not lend thee a penny."

As a creative writing student, I wondered what went into Shakespeare's thought process when he crafted Pistol's reply to that unfortunate news. So I accessed the bootlegged original notebooks of Shakespeare that I found on the dark web (the FBI subsequently shut down the site, so I can't point you to the source). It appears that Shakespeare struggled to choose between two responses when writing the play's first draft. This is what he considered:

Falstaff: "I will not lend thee a penny."

Pistol (*Response A*): "Why, then the world's mine oyster, which I with sword will open."

Pistol (*Response B*): "That doth bringeth sorrow to mine ears. I shall retreat to my bedchamber to slumber as a weary barnacle, clinging to the vessel of night. I pray thee, let the morrow bringeth a change of heart, for desperate be my hopes. Else, methinks I shall be shitteth out of luck."

Do you know which response Shakespeare selected? Reread them if you're unsure. It was *Response A*: "Why, then the world's mine oyster, which I with sword will open." With those stirring words, Pistol proclaimed he was empowered to acquire any of the world's bountiful offerings he wanted. And thus, the immortal phrase "the world is your oyster" entered our lexicon.

When you wake up each morning, the world can be your oyster. Or it can be your dried-up, stinky clam left rotting in the sun for two days. It is always up to you to decide how to seize the day, if at all.

Take a moment and think about what you did *last week*. Did you pry open the oyster and slurp to your heart's content, or did the week's promise slip through your fingers? How about *last year*? Did you live those precious twelve months like it was your final year on earth, or did you fall short of that lofty standard? Since we're in a provocative mood, how did you fare *last decade*? You had ten years on this beautiful, opportunity-soaked planet. Did you advance confidently in the direction of your dreams, or do you wish you could have a mulligan?

If you are like most of us, that thought exercise was eye-opening. You probably identified stuff you're doing right, but there were likely opportunities to take your life satisfaction to another level. You could have a hibernating dream that won't wake from its slumber. Your career may be unfulfilling, yet you're doing nothing about it. Maybe you need more adventure. Or you should commit to a healthier lifestyle. How are you leaving love on the table by not pursuing what your SAGe knows would fulfill you?

Wherever your gaps are, you're not alone. Others are experiencing the same challenges. Some take action to intentionally bring love into their life, while others succumb to the comforting sedation of excuses. Which camp do you want to pitch your tent in—the SAGe-inspired doers who take command of their lives and pursue their passions, or the excuse zombies?

The Wellness Ethic classifies your pursuits into three general categories:

○ *Personal Pursuits:* activities you engage in for enjoyment or personal enrichment rather than work or other responsibilities

○ *Professional Pursuits:* activities related to your career

○ *Lifestyle Maintenance (covered in chapter 18):* activities that help your life function, such as money management and household chores

To manifest a rewarding life, you should maintain a satisfying balance *across* the three categories (work-life balance) and find ways to get the most satisfaction out of your experiences *within* each category. Whatever you do, you want your experiences to be satisfaction-dense to optimize love, much like you want what you eat to be nutrient-dense to optimize your health. **A satisfaction-dense experience delivers a potent dose of love relative to the time and resources you put into it.** That love, which produces happiness and fulfillment, feeds your mind, body, and spirit.

Satisfaction-dense experiences are always within reach. You could be happy binge-watching a TV show with your partner because it relaxes you, and that's what you need at the moment. You could mindfully enjoy crocheting a blanket and getting lost in the craft of creating something beautiful from a string of yarn. Or you could feel fulfilled getting a professional certification, knowing that you are growing your skills and furthering your career.

When you live a SAGe-inspired life, you seek experiences that create love. The more you know yourself and what you love, the better you can guide your pursuits, whether those pursuits are planned or result from serendipity. Otherwise, it would be like following a broken compass in the wilderness and hoping to stumble upon an experience treasure.

Thankfully, you have already put in a lot of work getting underneath what's important to you. The My Compass tool you filled out in chapter

8—which identified your values, superpowers, ordered loves, and life purpose—will be a valuable resource in helping you determine what you want to pursue personally and professionally.

Let's get into this, starting with *personal pursuits.*

## Personal Pursuits

The pitted old sword with the dark patina grabbed my attention. It was a massive armament dating to the late 1200s to early 1300s, about when the last Crusade ended. It was in relic (dug from the ground) condition but was stable and fully intact. I had seen nearly a thousand antique swords over the years in the internet auctions I followed, but they were usually from the American Revolutionary War to the Civil War era. This sword on Heritage Auctions predated them by close to five hundred years. It had the wow factor. I really wanted it.

Unfortunately, the pre-auction estimated price range put it out of reach. But that was okay. I could still play my version of *The Price Is Right*: guess what I thought the sword would go for, track it during pre-auction bidding, and see what the hammer price was on auction day. I would enjoy that.

Before I logged off the Heritage website, I had to show the sword to my wife. She had developed an interest in history over the years (due to my influence), and I thought the sword would fascinate her. Perhaps she would love it so much that she would tell me to throw fiscal caution to the wind and go after it. Something like, "Mark, this pitted, medieval sword in relic condition is so damn cool! I want you to spend whatever it takes to obliterate the competition and win this auction! I must possess this sword!" She had never said anything remotely like that in the past when I coveted an out-of-reach collectible, but I always held out hope. In this case, she matter-of-factly said, "That sword is neat. Too bad it's so expensive." And then she went on her merry way, with no regard to my broken heart.

Yet I found the strength to carry on. I checked in on the sword every day. Scores of people were tracking it—it was one of the most popular lots in the auction—but no one had placed an absentee bid. That seemed odd. Usually, when an auction lot has this much interest, collectors jockey for position, and the bidding starts before the live auction. I thought there might be a possibility that people were curious about the sword but wouldn't bid. Not many militaria collectors pursue artifacts from the Middle Ages. Perhaps I had a chance—*Stop it, Mark. You're overthinking things. You're not getting the sword.*

Auction day arrived. I watched the live event online. When the sword was about to come up, I called my wife into my office so she could witness the bidding frenzy. The auctioneer introduced the sword. I typed in a modest bid but didn't hit "Enter." I looked at my wife for approval; she nodded. I didn't really expect to place the bid—I was just messing around—but okay, we're entering the arena! I placed the bid. I expected a flurry of activity to shoot up the price to at least triple what I had entered. Even if I were outbid by an increment, I would have to bow out. My bid was my upper limit.

But I didn't have to bow out because no one topped my bid! *Going, going, gone!* The hammer strikes—we win!

What a thoroughly enjoyable experience, not just on that day but also in the weeks preceding the auction and every day since. I love history. I love the stories. The character arcs. The inspiration. The wisdom. I enjoy thinking about how people lived in past eras. I read about history. I watch documentaries. I tour historical sites. I visit museums. And when given the opportunity, I collect history, which makes the past come alive. History is one of my great passions.

With the sword auction, I also enjoyed the intrigue of discovery and the thrill of the chase. After we won, I was happy as I anticipated the arrival of the sword shipment. I had fun determining how to fit the sword on one of my overcrowded walls (I also enjoy interior design despite my color blindness). Now that the sword is hung in its permanent spot in my office,

I get a tiny dopamine hit when I glance at it, a dopamine infusion when I mindfully engage, and I enjoy sharing the fascinating artifact with guests. History—and all the ways I bring it into my life—is a personal pursuit I love.

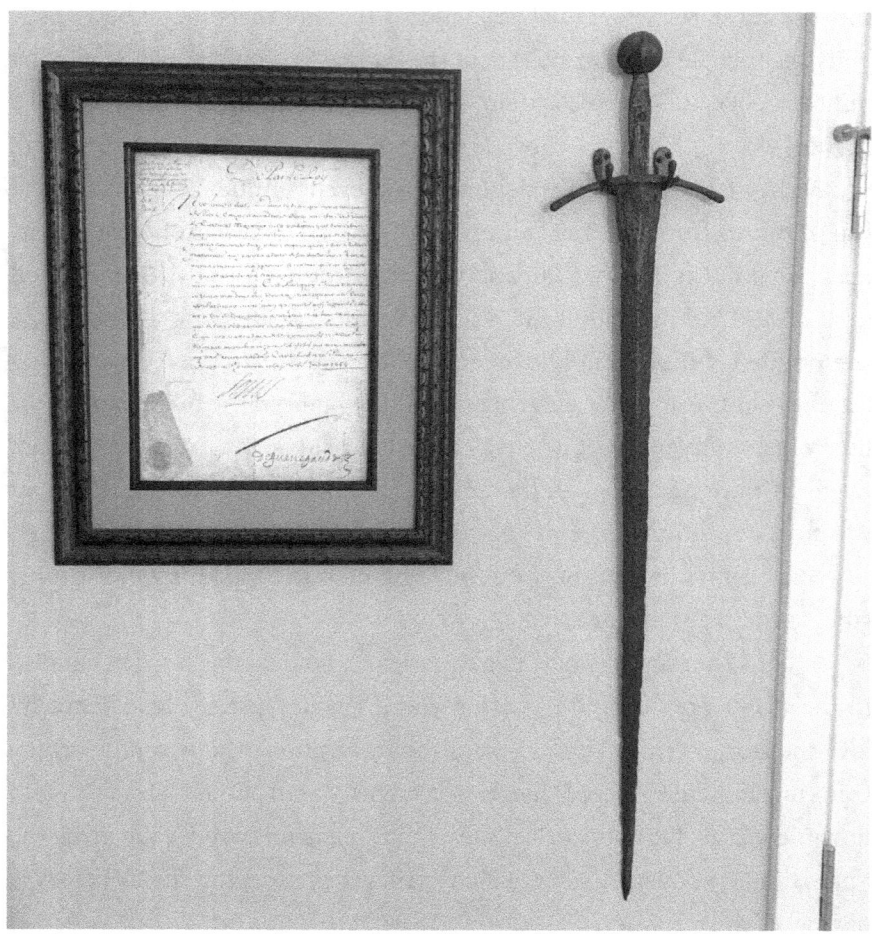

1665 King Louis XIV signed document / Medieval sword, late 1200s–early 1300s

You engage in personal pursuits for enjoyment or personal enrichment rather than to fulfill work or other responsibilities. The list of what you can pursue is only restricted by the limits of your imagination. You can enjoy playing sports, reading, watching movies, learning a language, volunteering, traveling, meditating, writing (provided you derive pleasure from pound-ing your head on your desk), socializing, gardening, collecting antiques, painting, cooking, fishing, playing video games . . .

Your level of engagement in the activity can be limited or, like history is for me, immersive. Whatever you do, and for however long you do it, you want to get the most out of the finite time and resources available to pursue your interests. You want your pursuits to be satisfaction-dense.

## Satisfaction-Dense Personal Pursuits

When you think about making your personal pursuits "satisfaction-dense," you may feel a twinge of dread and think: *Aren't we making this too complicated? Can't we just be?* Of course you can just be. When you seek satisfaction-dense experiences, there's no need to feel pressure to plan or optimize every minute of your day. That's not what it's about.

Satisfaction density is about flowing with the current of your life and getting the most out of your experiences. You may decide, at times, to be spontaneous, hop in a river, and see where the current takes you. Or you may intentionally create a satisfying experience by getting in a raft and steering it down the river—sometimes you'll choose a lazy river ride; other times, a white-water adventure. For this section, I'll focus on the times when you decide to be intentional with your personal pursuits.

There are many approaches to creating satisfaction-dense experiences in your personal life. We'll walk through some of them to get your mind inspired:

○ *Mindfully engage in what you do.* Deeply appreciate your partner throughout a date night and emotionally connect with why you love them. Take a nature walk and engage your senses with everything you encounter. Go to a restaurant and soak in the experience—the ambience, food, companionship, and the staff's hustle. Try to create a "flow" moment when engaging in a sport or a hobby.

○ *Increase the challenge with what you pursue—develop mastery.* Strive to set a personal record (PR) in an eighteen-round of golf (for me, a PR would be to hit fewer than four people with an errant golf ball). Visit every national park. Join a recreational sports league. Increase your charity fundraising target by 50%. Take classes in something that you love. Become a buff (Civil War, Disney, classic cars). Perfect your own brand of home brew.

○ *Diversify a pursuit.* Experiment with different kinds of meditation. Start a blog or a podcast around a passion. Read books from unfamiliar genres. Sample music or poetry from diverse cultures.

○ *Add other loves to a pursuit to multiply the love.* Instead of exercising by yourself, exercise with a friend. Take a dance class with your partner. Listen to a podcast on a subject you love as you do housework, drive, or go for a walk. Travel with a group of friends. Organize a charity softball tournament.

○ *Pursue something you have never done before.* Take scuba diving lessons. Volunteer in a foreign country. Go to an opera. Visit the Galapagos Islands. Learn how to play the bagpipes. Try a new water sport. Go to Burning Man. Learn how to paint. Start a garden.

I'll go through an example. Let's say you love food and want to get the most out of that pursuit by making it satisfaction-dense. You could take cooking classes. Prepare a five-course meal for friends. Participate in the *alphabet restaurant challenge* by going to a restaurant you have never frequented before that starts with the letter *A* and work your way to *Z*. Sell baked goods at a farmers' market. Learn how to cook food from a different culture each month. Take a vacation centered around your culinary interests, such as visiting famous BBQ joints in Kansas City. Have a mission to create the perfect cinnamon roll (a very worthy pursuit). Start a food blog.

Volunteer at a soup kitchen. What else could you do to get the most enjoyment out of your love for food?

With personal pursuits, the world is your oyster. How will you slurp that gift? Do you want to try something new? Something off the wall? Do you want to spend a Saturday afternoon losing yourself in a Ken Follett paperback? Or do you want to scale back on a current activity because it's not giving you enough joy? At the end of this chapter, we'll go through an exercise to determine where you want to take this. In the meantime, let's get down to business.

## Professional Pursuits

The ancient Greek philosopher Aristotle said, "Knowing yourself is the beginning of all wisdom." Clearly, he came up with that profound quote later in life and not when he was a high school numskull filling out a college application.

It was 1987, and I was staring at RPI's paper application. Getting past the drudgery was all that was between me and a pick-up basketball game. I zipped through the demographic section and then needed to select a major. No one had ever counseled me on how to approach that. I couldn't conduct online research—the internet wasn't in the public domain yet. I imagined a college major would lead to a career, so that seemed like a good place to start. What did I want to do after college? Become a lawyer? A social studies teacher? An exotic polka dancer? And which majors would lead me to one of those jobs?

I was clueless. At eighteen, I was experiencing my first mid-life crisis. *Can't I be done with this stupid form already?*

I went into speed-round mode as I scanned the list of options. Engineering and sciences? *Nope, too technical.* Architecture? *That would be cool, but I'm lousy with spatial relations.* Liberal arts? *What is that?* Business management?

*Seems practical—I could work for a corporation after graduation. All righty, business management it is!* I checked the box, completed the rest of the application, and then stuffed it into an envelope. I didn't realize that once I sealed the envelope, I would fight for over thirty years not to let that action seal my fate. But at least I got to play hoops that day!

It took me less than twenty seconds to choose a college major and a lifetime to try and undo it. If I had it to do all over again, I would have selected a course of study that led me down the path to becoming a psychologist, a filmmaker, a historian, a sports general manager, a venture capitalist, a writer, or an archaeologist. Occupations like that would have aligned better with my passions. But I can't change the past since time travel is a skill I have yet to master (it's next up on my to-do list after I solve a couple of quantum mechanics conundrums standing between me and the power of invisibility).

Once I graduated from RPI with a bachelor's degree in business management, I started my career in corporate America. I'll summarize the gory details: thirty years, six companies, four industries, five relocations, two coasts, six states, fifteen jobs, hundreds of talented colleagues, and three stupid layoffs.

The jobs ranged from individual contributor roles to executive positions leading departments. My specialty was business transformation, which involved applying strategic planning, change leadership, and Lean Six Sigma process improvement methodologies to drive business performance (it's what Waylon Jennings and Willie Nelson sang about in their chart-topping song, "Mammas, Don't Let Your Babies Grow Up to Be Business Transformation Professionals"). I haven't ascended to the C-suite yet, and probably never will, but I've carved out a respectable living that supports my family.

Unfortunately, there was never a single day I would have chosen to work in my corporate job if I didn't need the income. Though some aspects were fulfilling, my corporate career always fell short of what I required to be professionally satisfied. So I pursued side hustles to close the gap.

Working on side hustles has been a constant presence in my adult life. After college, I wrote screenplays for twenty years. I ran a part-time coaching business for a year. I helped launch an international consulting firm for another year. My social media start-up, Paloozoo, was active for four years. And I have devoted five years (so far) to writing this book. Over the years, I've spent about twenty hours a week on these efforts. This has been on top of working at my day job, being very involved with my family, exercising, and engaging in personal pursuits. Good Lord, this has been a grueling thirty years!

But I *needed* to do side hustles for my life to feel complete. They gave me autonomy to pursue opportunities that aligned with my life purpose. They challenged me and expanded my capabilities. I would have done them for free, but I also liked the potential to earn extra income.

Whether side hustles are right for you depends on your situation. No matter how you approach your professional pursuits, the more they align with your life purpose and what you love, the more satisfying your life will be.

## Professional Pursuits and Satisfaction Density

Professional pursuits are activities that you engage in related to your career. They include what you do in your job, of course, but they also encompass professional development opportunities like earning certifications and degrees, writing articles or books, and joining professional organizations.

Typically, the main outcome you seek from your professional pursuits is to fund your lifestyle. But when you consider that most working people dedicate nearly half their waking hours to their job (including commute time), you'll also want your work to satisfy you. **Getting the most satisfaction out of your professional pursuits is synonymous with nurturing the wonderful gift of your existence.** Yes, all roads lead to satisfaction density!

To bring satisfaction density to your professional pursuits, you can:

○ *Mindfully engage in what you do.* Try to create "flow" when working on a task. Closely observe meeting dynamics (nonverbal cues, how people interact, momentum shifts, energy levels) and use those insights to influence the meeting outcomes. Practice deep breathing to increase focus before working on a project. Don't multitask.

○ *Increase the challenge with what you pursue—develop mastery.* Complete a task in half the time without sacrificing quality or safety. Set a stretch objective requiring you to expand your capabilities. Stay on top of industry trends. Practice to build mastery. Pursue certifications and degrees. Go to conferences. Use your superpowers to excel at your job. Work with your leader and human resources to develop a career path. Seek promotions or challenging lateral moves.

○ *Diversify a pursuit.* Start a blog around your area of expertise. Write a book or an article. Be a podcast guest. Present at a conference. Teach what you know. Offer your skills to a nonprofit.

○ *Add other loves to a pursuit to multiply the love.* Listen to podcasts and audiobooks related to your career while you do personal activities. Bring your child (or pet) to your workplace. Exercise while you take virtual meetings. Schedule meditation into your workday.

○ *Pursue something you have never done before.* Learn how to code. Job shadow in a different department. Design an app. Explore a career change. Volunteer to take on assignments outside your comfort zone.

Note: I have a list of 261 other ways you can feel satisfied in your professional pursuits, no matter what you do. But I won't overwhelm you here. They'll be included in this book's sequel, tentatively titled *The Wellness Ethic II: Theoretical Applications of Wellness Concepts to the Artificial Lives of Androids and Other Mechanical Contraptions.* I'll release the book once robots take over the planet.

Doesn't this professional stuff seem easy? You just land a job that pays well, develop your skills as you go, and find ways to make work interesting. But don't forget that it would be awesome to do a job you love that aligns with your life purpose ... And you want to accomplish meaningful stuff ... And live a balanced life ... And not be flattened by disruption ...

I can't believe you fell into my trap! No, this career stuff ain't easy! It wasn't even easy five hundred years ago! In the 1500s, you would have dealt with wagonloads of disruption as you tried to eke out a living. I'll list a few sixteenth-century disruptors in case you yearn for simpler times: the bubonic plague, wars, witch hunts, famines, the Americas, smallpox, the Religious Reformation—hold your horses, I'm just getting warmed up!

Managing a career in the twenty-first century is challenging because your professional life is an unpredictable, ever-evolving journey that's prone to disruption. There's that "D" word again—*disruption*. Disruption is fracturing our professional bedrock. It warrants a deeper dive.

## Thrive Professionally in a Disruptive World

I can't tell you what the future of work will look like in five years or even next month. The list of work disruptors is dizzying. Here are a few:

○ *AI and Automation*: The artificial intelligence (AI) technologies that automate routine and repetitive tasks continue to disrupt careers. As capabilities advance, AI will climb the food chain and automate more complex tasks. This will eliminate jobs and create others.

○ *Competition*: Low barriers to entry and the rapid rate of innovation create competitive disruption, which can impact a company's fortunes overnight.

○ *Trends in HR and Organizational Design*: A drive for efficiency affects organizational structure. Remote/hybrid/in-office work policies continue to evolve. High demand for skilled talent creates opportunity.

○ *Economy/Stock Market*: In a bear market, companies contract, and layoffs occur; in a bull market, companies grow, and jobs are created.

○ *Globalization*: The world is a global economy, and companies will continue to move work to lower-cost countries and leverage international talent (especially with technology making it easy to perform virtual work).

○ *Gig Economy*: The gig economy, which involves short-term contracts and freelance work, provides opportunities for people to start businesses or work as contractors, but it can also create more competition for traditional jobs.

No one can accurately predict how the intersection of these disruptors will play out. And I didn't even include disruptors like geopolitical forces, climate change, government policy, pandemics, or immigration!

The future of work is uncertain—blah, blah, blah—we knew that already! When we think about career disruption, it's helpful to consider the Japanese concept of *ikigai*, which represents the intersection of what you love, what you are good at, what the world needs, and what you can get paid for. When those elements harmonize in your professional life, you are fulfilled.

But disruption can throw them off-kilter. You may find that you're good at something the world no longer needs (or needs less of) because technology has satisfied the demand. A new career can be created from disruption that excites you, but your skills may not align (unless you do something about it!). Your pay could go up or down based on disruptive influences. If *ikigai* is jumbled in your life, how can you restore order? Hint: Applying the Accept-Frame-Respond model would be a great place to start as you build your plan.

Though you can't always predict how or when disruption will occur, you can still position yourself for the best outcome—that's all you can control.

Let's make this more real. Think about your job—or one that you want to hold—and consider how disruption could impact it. Try envisioning your professional future over the next three to five years (or beyond). Contemplate how disruption could impact your profession and your company.

Mind-numbing, isn't it? As is happening now and will continue in the future, some jobs will become obsolete, others will be created, and all careers will evolve. That's not intended to strike fear in your heart. It's just reality.

*But it's okay.* We're on a Wellness Ethic journey, so we surrender to the ways of the universe and accept that disruption is real. We use our growth mindset to select an optimistic frame that we'll find a way to adapt. Our empowered SAGe then chooses a proactive response that flows with the white-water rapids and puts us in the best position to thrive professionally.

With the 80/20 rule in mind, there are six principles I'll share that can position you to thrive professionally in the unpredictable world of disruption: *(1) know the professional you, (2) nurture a productive mindset, (3) take care of business today, (4) cultivate your network, (5) be forward thinking,* and *(6) take action to position for tomorrow.* These principles will get you thinking about possibilities, but that's just a start. The real work will be executing a plan to transform that potential into your reality. This is all in your wheelhouse!

## PRINCIPLE #1: **KNOW THE PROFESSIONAL YOU**

The more you're intimate with what satisfies you professionally (the My Compass tool in chapter 8 will help), the better you can steer your career in a rewarding direction. Reflect upon the following questions to uncover the "professional you" (consider documenting your answers):

*How does your career align with your values (My Compass)?* When your career aligns with your values, you are motivated. When it doesn't, the spiritual disconnect often leads to dissatisfaction and disengagement.

*How does your career align with your superpowers (My Compass)?* When you use your gifts at work, you're doing what you were created to do. You tend to excel at your job and your satisfaction and self-esteem rise.

*How does your career align with your ordered loves (My Compass)?* A career can align with your passions, but it can also, at times, take you away from what you love the most. Do you love your job?

*How does your career align with your life purpose (My Compass)?* A career on purpose provides fulfilling opportunities to create love and positively impact the world. A fulfilling career can be a vital part of a well-lived life.

*What do you like to do that satisfies you professionally?* Examples: leadership, service, creativity, engineering, analysis, coding, problem-solving, teaching, working in specific industries . . .

*What don't you like professionally?* Examples: tedious tasks, micromanagement, overwork, specific work schedules, high stress, limited autonomy, lack of meaning . . .

*What are your professional strengths?* Examples: learning, leadership, creativity, technical skills, industry or job experience, problem-solving, communication, emotional intelligence, service, strategic thinking, execution . . .

*What outcomes do you want out of your career?* Examples: job satisfaction, money and benefits, achievement, growth, positive work environment, social connection, realizing your life purpose, security, skill mastery, being part of a mission . . .

At the end of this chapter, I included an exercise to help you identify the five most important factors, in rank order, that define the "professional you" and drive your professional satisfaction. Your SAGe can use that list to guide your career along a fulfilling path.

### PRINCIPLE #2: **NURTURE A PRODUCTIVE MINDSET**

In a disruptive climate, your happiness is at risk as your career can seem like it's targeted by a sledgehammer in a game of whack-a-job. But, as you know, negativity stymies growth and greatly diminishes your chances of success.

Conversely, a productive mindset creates positive energy. You become happier and more motivated as your SAGe fully activates to meet the disruptive moment.

There are six productive mindsets that are especially powerful when faced with disruption. Adopting these mindsets gives you an edge in life, not only in your professional pursuits but in all pursuits, during times of turmoil and times of stability.

○ *Growth Mindset:* When you have a growth mindset, you believe that your abilities can develop over time. You view disruption as an opportunity to learn and grow. You seek new experiences.

○ *Positive Mindset:* A person with a positive attitude has an optimistic outlook that things will work out, even during challenging times. They approach disruption with a "can-do" energy.

○ *Stoic Mindset:* A Stoic focuses on what they can control—their thoughts and actions—and avoids getting consumed by negativity resulting from circumstances out of their control, like disruption.

○ *Proactive Mindset:* A proactive person anticipates and addresses challenges before they arise and takes action to prevent them from worsening if they do occur.

○ *Resilient Mindset:* When you are resilient, you're motivated to move forward despite challenges and setbacks. You have a stubborn tenacity to persevere in the face of adversity.

○ *Flexible Mindset:* A flexible person adapts to disruption by being open to new ideas and embracing different ways of doing things.

To adopt these mindsets, review the techniques in chapters 4 and 6 and apply the ones that resonate. You could: (1) keep your intention to adopt the mindsets in front of you through positive journaling, affirmations, and visual management, (2) put the Accept-Frame-Respond model through the productive mindsets lens when choosing a response to disruption, and (3) seek support through life coaching or mentoring.

## PRINCIPLE #3: **TAKE CARE OF BUSINESS TODAY**

Having professional objectives and a plan to get there is good. But first things first: Take care of business today by ensuring you're fully engaged in your current job and making an impact. Your job performance influences your job security, pay, professional growth, the respect you have within your network (which can lead to opportunities), and even your happiness. Though it's never a perfect science—life isn't always fair—people who make the greatest impact at work tend to get rewarded more than those who deliver less.

To "take care of business today" also means getting as much satisfaction as possible from your job by engaging in satisfaction-dense opportunities. How can you grow professionally by increasing the challenge of your work and expanding your capabilities? Which aspects of your role are enjoyable and fulfilling? If possible, try to include more of those activities in your job to boost your satisfaction and get better results for your company and customers.

For example, I've led business transformation functions in my career and am passionate about positive leadership and strategic planning. So rest assured, if you're ever in an organization I lead (I'll apologize in advance for your career misfortune), we'll have an identity as a team that centers around positive leadership—it'll become our team brand. We'll also have a vision and growth strategy for how our team impacts our company's results and boosts its culture. That stuff is never in my job description, but I still do it. It's impactful, and I need to be satisfied in my job.

Job satisfaction is also dependent upon addressing job dissatisfaction. Do any of your job activities or responsibilities dissatisfy you? Try to minimize the dissatisfaction as much as possible. For instance, you can reduce unnecessary meetings or eliminate tasks that don't add value. Is a coworker creating friction? Work with the person to resolve the conflict and build a productive relationship, or involve your manager or human resources to facilitate a resolution. The more dissatisfaction you remove from your job, the more room you'll have for satisfaction-dense activities. You'll also be happier.

Everything we've covered with "taking care of business" relies on your engagement with your work. However, fully engaging in a job is sometimes challenging when you don't love what you do. But don't accept that excuse. Instead, consider your job's noble purpose and let it inspire you. Your job can provide money to support your family. It can provide value to customers and society. It can develop your skills and grow your experience.

Here are examples of a job's noble purpose: A hairdresser is an artist who makes their clients feel beautiful. A lawyer represents clients overwhelmed by the legal system who need help to serve their vital interests. An Uber driver provides a cost-effective and safe transportation service to help passengers live satisfying lives. What is the noble purpose of your job?

## PRINCIPLE #4: CULTIVATE YOUR NETWORK

A diverse network can help you deepen your knowledge about your profession and what the future may hold. It can open your mind to possibilities beyond your current career path. Your network can also be a sounding board, provide mentorship, lend support, offer exposure, and refer job leads.

Cultivating mutually beneficial relationships with people who align with your professional interests is one of the keys to thriving in the age of disruption. To build your network, connect with colleagues within your company, engage with online platforms like LinkedIn, attend industry events and other gatherings, and get introductions to people through your family, friends, and professional connections. Basically, every time you interact with someone, it presents an opportunity to grow your network.

When you branch out and interact with other professionals, your horizons expand, which can translate into career growth and future opportunities. Not only does a network contribute to your career prospects, but the camaraderie you nurture can be one of the most fun and fulfilling aspects of your professional life.

PRINCIPLE #5: **BE FORWARD THINKING**

What will your profession look like in the future? Which disruption-friendly career paths align with what you love to do, even if they represent career shifts? To expand your knowledge of the future, you can conduct online research, ask people in your company and network for their perspectives, read articles and books, listen to podcasts, and utilize other resources.

At this exploratory stage, it's critical that you nurture a productive mindset. Don't let limiting beliefs close your mind or crush your enthusiasm. You can always develop new skills. You have unlimited capabilities and potential. Career pivots are always possible. The world is your oyster. These aren't just hollow words in a paragraph in a wellness book—*they represent your truth.*

If you struggle with motivation at this stage, a thought-provoking question that can inspire your productive mindset is: How can disruption become a professional "win" for you? Summon your SAGe and intentionally apply the productive mindsets we covered to shift your mindset away from viewing disruption as a threat but rather as a compelling opportunity to do something exciting that aligns with your life purpose and what you love. Find the gift in disruption.

Based on your forward-thinking, fact-finding mission, what would it take to pursue a disruption-friendly career path that interests you? Do you need to develop specific skills and experiences? Or get a certification? Do you need to expand your network and connect with people aligned with your career interests? Do you need exposure? The path forward may seem overwhelming, but that's why a SAGe breaks down their intentions into manageable steps, which leads us to the next principle:

### PRINCIPLE #6: **TAKE ACTION TO POSITION FOR TOMORROW**

To succeed in your career, it's essential to embrace the dual focus of work: getting your job done well today while you position yourself for a rewarding tomorrow. Keeping those balls up in the air requires an intentional approach.

To pursue a disruption-friendly career path, what can you do today, next week, next month, and beyond to position for success? To build out your plan, a starting point can be to follow the *Why? – Define – Position – Do* steps in chapter 6. Determine your why, define your objectives, build a plan and a change adoption approach, and then execute.

A primary focus of your plan will likely be a learning strategy shaped by your growth mindset. In a disruptive world, continuous learning is how you surf the wave of change. As you develop your learning strategy, consider building expertise in skills that will be in demand as disruption occurs. That approach doesn't just extend to technical skills within your profession but also to skills that are transferable to practically any profession, such as leadership, problem-solving, communications, technology proficiency, and creativity.

Your skills and past experiences serve you, no matter which career direction you take. Nothing is ever wasted. Skills and experiences are building blocks that give you a foundation to handle whatever crosses your professional path. And when you encounter something new that your foundation isn't fully prepared to handle, then add more blocks to your foundation by seeking help and developing new skills and experiences! That's what people do to build thriving careers.

A career will challenge you (you wouldn't want it any other way). It will be unpredictable. There will be ups and downs. Stupid things will happen.

The job you have today is never guaranteed to be permanent. In fact, the odds are very, very strong that it won't be. Career pivots will be necessary.

Sometimes, you may need to take a step back from a compensation or job-level standpoint—one step back to take two steps forward—to execute a career pivot. But through it all, keep your eye on the prize: You want to feel and share love in everything you do, including your professional pursuits. By doing so, you will be satisfied. You will have honored your values and life purpose. You will have nurtured the wonderful gift of your existence.

## Case Study—Customer Service Representative

Tara works as a customer service rep at a software company. She worries about losing her job as chatbots automate more and more of her role.

*Tara's Response*: Tara was always wise to take care of business at her current job. She performs at an "exceeds level," has built a good network, and is known for having a passion for helping customers. She wants to stay with the software company and work directly with product development. However, she is concerned that her lack of technology experience could hold her back.

Tara talks with her manager, human resources, and members of her trusted network about her career interests. They bring up the possibility of working as a requirements analyst (a job that creates and documents software design requirements) or a quality assurance analyst (a job that tests software products). Both product-related positions would leverage Tara's technical experience in helping customers resolve product issues and could be a great way to start a career in the product and technology space. She loves the idea.

To move forward, Tara builds out a plan, with her leader's support, to job shadow employees in those roles, work on future projects that will give her relevant experience, attend training classes to build expertise, and pursue a degree in computer science (the company will reimburse part of the cost). Earning a degree will require a significant time and financial commitment, but after discussing it with her partner, they agree that it will serve their long-term interests to make the sacrifice. Her partner supports her so she can get to "yes."

By taking charge of her career with a growth mindset, Tara focused on what she could control—her attitude and actions. She responded proactively to disruption and put herself in the best position for a thriving career.

**With personal and professional pursuits, the world is your oyster—so pig out on mollusks!**

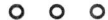

## Move Forward on Your Wellness Ethic Journey!

① **Personal Pursuits:** Using your My Compass tool as a guide, document what you want to focus on with your personal pursuits.

<br><br><br><br>

② **Professional Pursuits:** Fill in the chart to get underneath what drives your professional satisfaction. For your satisfaction drivers, list them in rank order and then rate how you are performing with each one in your current job (use a scale of 1 to 5, with 1 = "poorly" and 5 = "very well").

| Top 5 Drivers of My Professional Satisfaction | Score |
|---|---|
| 1 | |
| 2 | |
| 3 | |
| 4 | |
| 5 | |
| Improvement & Change Adoption Focus | |
| | |

③ Advanced Topics (going beyond the 80/20): Research how artificial intelligence could impact your professional life. Develop a strategy to adapt based on what you discover.

# Mark's Example

(1) **Personal Pursuits:** Using your My Compass tool as a guide, document what you want to focus on with your personal pursuits.

> I'll plan trips with my wife to visit our children—a trip to Denver, Colorado, and one to Gainesville, Florida. It will be a great opportunity to spend time with family and experience mountains, parks, and tasty cuisine. Perfect satisfaction density!

(2) **Professional Pursuits:** Fill in the chart to get underneath what drives your professional satisfaction. For your satisfaction drivers, list them in rank order and then rate how you are performing with each one in your current job (use a scale of 1 to 5, with 1 = "poorly" and 5 = "very well").

| | Top 5 Drivers of My Professional Satisfaction | Score |
|---|---|---|
| 1 | Earn money and benefits to support my family | 4 |
| 2 | Work aligns with my life purpose and is impactful | 2.5 |
| 3 | Achieve a healthy work-life balance | 3.5 |
| 4 | Leverage my leadership and creative talents | 2.5 |
| 5 | Have autonomy with the focus of my work | 2 |

### Improvement & Change Adoption Focus

I want to explore what it would take to leave corporate America and focus full-time on writing my book. What would that do to my family's ability to make ends meet? What risk would we be assuming? What impact would that have on retirement? Finishing this book and being able to put all of my energy into it is very important to me—it aligns with my life purpose. I'll commit to doing the analysis and planning to see what's feasible.

# Lifestyle Maintenance

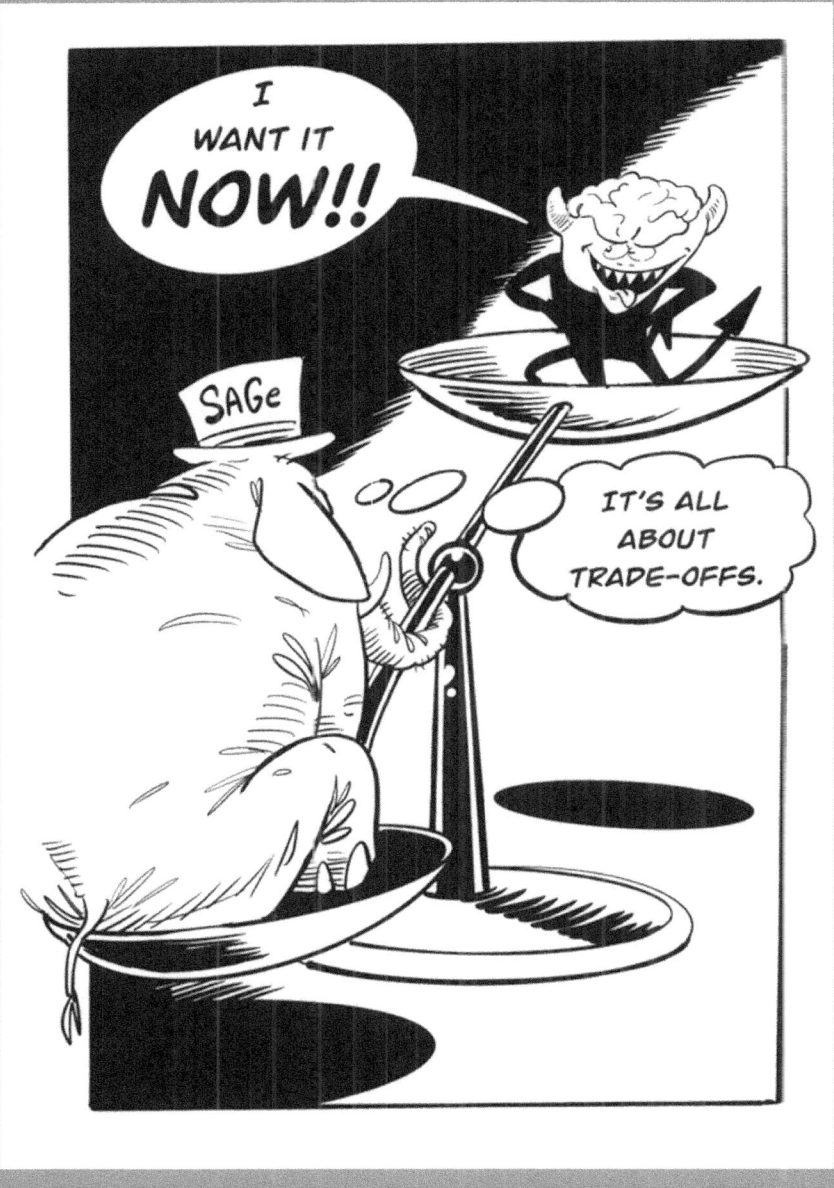

# CHAPTER 17

# A Story of Gratitude

There's something magical about buying your first home.

After you complete the closing process and have your keys, you drive to your house. You can't wait to step inside. You've been there before, but it was always rushed, with a real estate agent trailing your every move. You never got a true sense of the house and its energy. *What is the layout again?*

When you arrive at your new home, you march to the front door and insert the key. The door opens. *Phew.* It would have really sucked if it didn't. You would have had to drive back to the closing attorney's office—if they're still open—and see if they gave you the wrong key. If they can't help, you may have to call a locksmith. It would be a setback to your special day. But thankfully, the door opened, so you don't have to deal with all that crap.

You enter your house and explore. You go to every room, look out every window, open every closet. Then it hits you. You are the master of your domain. You can make renovations, grow a garden, and decorate your house in a style that brings you joy, even if that joy comes from hanging your beloved *Velvet Elvis* painting in the dining room. I'm not here to judge.

Moving into a home is a new beginning. Whether it's an apartment or a house, whether you rent or buy, or the place is big or small, you can make it your own. What do you love? What inspires you? What are your values? Your home can reflect who you are and bring happiness into your life.

My wife, Kristen, and I bought our first house in 1994 when our daughter Audrey was a toddler. We could afford the house thanks to a government first-time home buyer's program and support from my grandfather, who helped with the $5,000 down payment. It was a newly constructed, two-story starter home in Mechanicville, New York (near Albany), around 1,300 square feet. It may have seemed small to some people, but it was a palace to us.

Over a few years, with the help of our extended family's home improvement know-how, we customized the house to get it just right, including finishing a basement that Kristen used to run a daycare business. The last major project was putting a roof on our deck and screening it. Thanks to my father, we finished that, and it looked great.

I can remember sitting on the deck in the evening with my wife after the project was complete. She was flying out to Colorado the next day with Audrey for a weeklong vacation to see her relatives. We were in a sentimental mood, and I remarked how fortunate we were to have our house. It was a modest home, but it fit our needs perfectly. Life was good.

After Kristen and Audrey left for Colorado, I had the week to myself. And no, the Reinisch homestead didn't become party central. There were no parties. No visitors. Just me and our three cats.

But the house did get quite messy due to my immature failure to recognize the value of a radical concept called "clean as you go." My family was coming back at 5:00 p.m. on a Saturday, so I planned to take that day to pull my house back from the precipice of being condemned.

Saturday arrived. I woke up at 7:00 a.m.—I couldn't wait to see my family. I had ten hours before their return. Everything had to be perfect for their homecoming, so I put on my game face—it was time to get busy!

I started with the interior—vacuuming, mopping, washing dishes, doing laundry, dusting, and cleaning bathrooms. I had a blast listening to music and plowing through the chores. By having so much to do in so little time, I had unintentionally created a gamified challenge.

After the interior was sparkling, I went grocery shopping. When I returned home, I put everything away except for a box of Hostess Chocolate

CupCakes (Kristen's favorite) and a bag of M&M's (Audrey's favorite) that I placed on the countertop. I then set up a vase with fresh flowers and centered it on the kitchen table. I wanted my family to know they were adored.

Next up was the exterior. It looked like rain was on the horizon, so I needed to hurry. I did the yard work in record time and straightened up the deck. Everything looked good, and I beat the storm! But the sky was dark and had a greenish hue that looked ominous. Whatever.

I walked into my house, removed my sweaty shirt and grass-stained socks, and grabbed a Sam Adams from the fridge. I popped open the beer and sat down at the kitchen table. I had pulled it off. Soon, I'd be getting big hugs from my family!

I finished the beer. It was time to take a shower. I walked to the stairs that would take me up to the main bathroom on the second story. Before ascending, I glanced toward my family room windows—the storm had arrived and was creating a stir. I strolled to the window to get a closer look. I was mesmerized by an old, thick pine tree in my backyard, struggling mightily as its branches swirled in the forceful wind. A large tree shouldn't move like that.

*I better shut the kitchen windows so the rain doesn't get in.*

I hurried to the kitchen. The casement window sash was getting caught in the wind, which made it shake. I turned the crank to shut the window, but it wouldn't budge. I tried again—no luck. The wind was too strong. Suddenly, the window sash flew off the hinge and smashed into the side of our garage—

*What the hell! This is gonna cost me a fortune to replace!*

The rain formed a puddle on the countertop.

*I've gotta get a towel.*

The towels were upstairs. I speed-walked toward the stairs and glanced again at the pine tree through the family room windows. It didn't look good—the wind had intensified. So I jogged to the window to get a closer look. The tree trunk was swaying, its branches twisting as if it were in a death match with Mother Nature.

*My God! This tree could snap!*

That was the last thought that entered my mind. I stopped thinking at the conscious level. Everything I did now was instinctual.

I ran back to the kitchen windows. Rain was drenching the countertop.

I ran to the stairs to get the towel on the second floor.

But something compelled me to turn and run into the family room to see what was happening to the pine tree. When I looked outside, I knew the tree was a second or two away from crashing down. PURE FEAR zapped every cell in my body! My senses were overwhelmed. I didn't think or hear anything or even recognize my fear. There was no time. I just found myself sprinting in a mad dash to my basement!

I reached the basement door and bounded down the stairs.

I got to the basement level. My heart was pounding!

I paced for about ten seconds to calm down and then noticed light shining through a foot-sized hole in the ceiling. I looked up through the hole—I could see the sky. My brain tried to process that bizarre anomaly.

*I shouldn't be able to see the sky through my basement ceiling. I have two stories of my house over that hole.*

Bewildered, I walked to my basement stairwell to get upstairs to check things out. I could only get halfway up—the stairwell was caved in.

*This makes no sense. There should be more stairs and a door. Why can't I go upstairs?*

Nothing was registering; I was shell-shocked. I walked to an oversized basement window and peered outside. My eyes were drawn to our screened deck. The deck's roof and walls were no longer there—only the deck floor remained.

*Ah, Jesus. I'll have to rebuild that. What's going on!?*

I walked back to the stairwell, hoping that I had imagined things. The stairwell was still impassable. I walked to the hole in my basement ceiling. I could still see the sky. I walked to my basement window and looked out. There still was no screened deck.

*What the hell has happened?*

I don't know if five minutes or thirty minutes passed—everything was a blur—but I soon heard a guy holler outside the window, "Is anyone in there?"

His voice jolted me out of my brain fog. "Yes, yes!" I shouted as I hurried to the window.

Three neighbors stood outside, peering into my basement. "We have to break the window to get you out," one of them said in a raised voice

"No! Don't do that!" I didn't want to have to replace the window.

"It's the only way you're getting out!"

"Okay! Let me step back!" I took a few steps back and turned away.

They smashed the window and cleared the glass.

I stepped onto a couch under the window. With their help, I pulled myself up through the opening. I was now outside.

I stood up and surveyed my property and neighborhood. Everything now made perfect sense. Finally!

My family no longer had a home.

A tornado had ripped through my neighborhood and reduced my two-story house to rubble. Tornadoes didn't happen in Mechanicville, New York. But one did on May 31, 1998, at 4:22 p.m., and it leveled our home. With me in it. And our three cats. And all of my family's valued possessions.

Nothing could have prepared my family for the aftermath of dealing with this disaster. The only thing we could do was take it step by step: start the insurance process, find a temporary place to live, sift through the rubble to see if anything was salvageable, and, most importantly, find our cats.

The ensuing days were a process of driving to the pile of debris that used to be our home, recovering what we could, and calling for our cats. But our beloved pets were nowhere to be found. *Maybe they had miraculously survived and were in the wild? Or—no, banish the thought of "or."*

After five days of sorting through the rubble and searching the basement (which was flooded with three feet of water due to a broken water pipe), we made one last trip to our house in hopes of finding our cats. The next day, the National Guard was scheduled to use heavy machinery to clear the property. We searched the site and called out their names—*Winston, JJ, Bamm-Bamm*. But there was no sign of them. We gave up hope. It was time to leave.

My wife headed to our minivan. I peered inside our basement window one last time and called out to them. A few seconds passed. Nothing. I was about to leave, but then I heard a faint *meow*!

I lowered myself through the broken window to the flooded basement. Within five minutes, I miraculously found all three cats scattered throughout the basement on boxes and shelves. They were safe and sound! It was one of the happiest moments of my life.

The tornado experience showed me that life is fragile. Possessions are temporary. Nothing you have is an entitlement. All the blessings that come your way can be taken away in the blink of an eye. **Don't ever take things for granted.**

I only feel profound gratitude when I think about the tornado today. I survived! It blows my mind how close I came to being unable to write those words. I would have died if I had completed my chores minutes earlier. The tornado wouldn't have been near when I glanced at the pine tree on my way upstairs, so the tree wouldn't have been twisting—it wouldn't have drawn my interest. I would have continued to the second story and been in the shower when my house crumbled. Or if I had delayed running into my basement by a couple of seconds, I would have been crushed to death by my collapsing home. There were so many close calls and so many instinctual decisions that saved my life.

But that's just the beginning of my gratitude. I am grateful that Kristen and Audrey weren't home when the tornado destroyed our house. I am grateful that we found our cats alive. I am grateful we had good insurance through State Farm and could rebuild our lives with the help of the settlement and the loving support of our family and friends. I am SO GRATEFUL that I have been blessed to be Kristen's husband and Audrey and Emma's father for decades after the tornado. I won't ever take that for granted.

Possessions can be replaced. Family, friends, and pets? They're a gift from the universe that should be treasured.

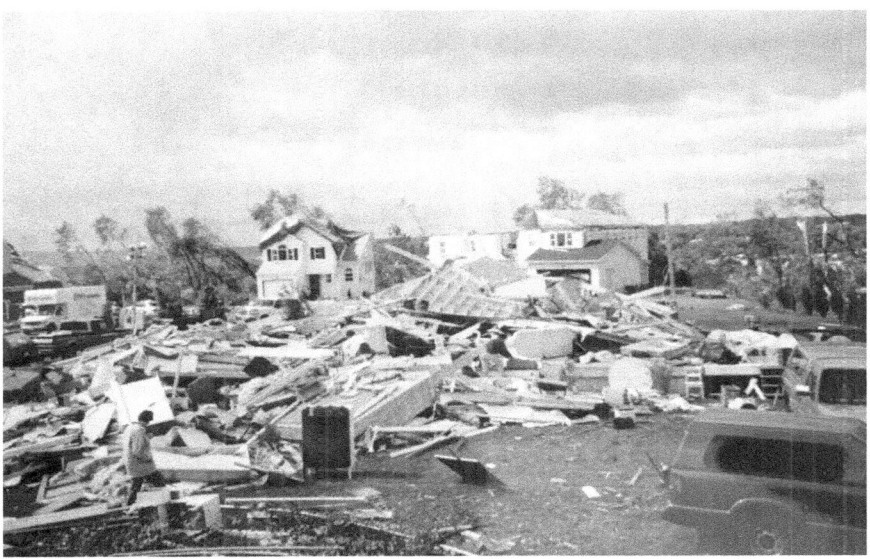

Our house—June 1998

o  o  o

# CHAPTER 18

# Maintain Your Life Better Than Your Yard

To write and publish *The Wellness Ethic* requires considerable time, which is a limited resource for me. I have many competing priorities that cry out "me, me, me, me, me." Some are sympathetic to my plight; many are not.

In addition to my book project, I devote time to my family and corporate job. I sleep and exercise. I engage in my mindfulness habit. I have fun. I also do tasks to maintain my lifestyle, such as completing house chores and managing money.

Lifestyle maintenance doesn't inspire me. But if I neglect it, my life will fall apart. I tend to my finances to pay the bills and retire someday. I take my cats to the vet because I love the little hooligans and they deserve to be healthy. I get my hair cut every few months so wild animals won't flock to me. But I can't accept lifestyle maintenance being a drag on my life. I need to nurture the wonderful gift of my existence in everything I do.

Our challenge in this chapter is determining how to maintain our lives as efficiently and effectively as possible while boosting our satisfaction. We shouldn't settle for less.

Applying the 80/20 rule, I'll break up lifestyle maintenance into two topics: *financial wellness* and *the annoying stuff* (chores, etc.).

# Financial Wellness

In 2008, during the Great Recession, I thought I would take advantage of the crashing stock market to make a quick buck—I have always been a fan of easy money. So I tried my hand at speculative investing and bought Washington Mutual (WaMu) stock. They were a large financial institution whose stock had plummeted below $5 a share. They were due for a huge rebound.

An alternate investment option I had considered was purchasing an Alexander Hamilton autographed letter from 1798. The letter shared Hamilton's plans to become Inspector General under George Washington during the Quasi-War with France. From a financial standpoint, the letter would appreciate over time, and personally, I would be delighted to see it framed on my office wall.

But in my super-sophisticated, savvy investor mind, I knew that WaMu's stock price would recover and triple my investment in a year or two. Besides, it wasn't like some guy was going to write a Broadway musical about Hamilton and boost the value of his memorabilia. Though my heart was with Hamilton, investing in WaMu was the responsible choice.

Soon after I made my surefire WaMu investment, they went belly-up. I lost every dollar I invested. Argh! The WaMu experience was a humbling wake-up call—my superpowers didn't extend to outwitting Wall Street.

I find that everything about money is hard. Except for spending it. Earning it is hard. Understanding investment options is hard. Developing a financial plan and sticking to it is hard. But here's the saving grace: You don't have to be a money wizard to move forward with financial wellness. If you understand your financial needs and translate those insights into a sensible plan that you follow, you can take control of your financial well-being. And there are experts and resources that can help you every step along the way—many are free. **You and I have the capability to be smart and disciplined with our money.**

When you assess the state of your finances, you could be thriving, doing okay, or living paycheck to paycheck. If you're in a rut, you may feel hopeless. But that's a limiting belief. Others have overcome the challenges you're facing. You can do the same. You can't change the past, but you are always empowered to apply your growth mindset to meet any challenge. You are always empowered to trust your SAGe to move your life forward.

Financial wellness is a journey you take step by step. It often begins slowly: You build a plan, adjust your saving and spending habits, accumulate wins, and learn from setbacks. By staying committed to your ever-evolving plan (life happens), money soon becomes an enabler of your well-being.

Financial wellness refers to the state of having control over your finances, including meeting your current and future financial needs, while maintaining a healthy mindset toward your financial situation. Before we dig deeper, I'll clear up two common misconceptions about money:

○ *False Belief #1: Money is a measuring stick of life success.* A rich person isn't successful because of that fact. Life success is a function of feeling and sharing love. Not money. I've known rich people who were rock stars at growing their bank accounts, and you literally couldn't pay me a billion dollars to live their lives. They were obsessed with money and status and never figured out how to be happy.

○ *False Belief #2: Happiness requires money.* Not true. Most things that make you happy cost very little, if anything. Spending time with loved ones. Sports. Nature. Volunteering. Reading. Laughing. Listening to music (unless it's going to a Taylor Swift concert; you'll need a second mortgage for that). Money is not the key to your happiness. How you perceive and respond to your world is what makes you happy.

Money isn't a cure-all for whatever ails you. But it can play a role in your wellness. It can support your basic needs, lifestyle, and pursuits. It can reduce stress as you worry less about making ends meet or being positioned for retirement. It can provide a safety net for when stupid things happen. Money can be a positive force in your life *when it stays centered around enabling well-being.*

That's what we'll focus on now—how to move forward in the direction of financial wellness to support a person's well-being. But I will need to be very modest in my 80/20 approach. I would do my readers a disservice if I attempted to provide a prescriptive path to financial well-being. Financial wellness is a broad subject that includes budgeting, debt management, investment strategies, retirement planning, and much more—a single chapter wouldn't do it justice. Financial wellness is also a journey that should be customized to your needs, preferably with the help of certified experts.

However, I will offer three basic steps to get you started on the right path: *know your financial guiding principles, leverage resources to build a financial plan*, and *be an active manager of your money.* For those already well-versed in these topics, the rest of this section can provide quick validation that you have the bases covered.

## Know Your Financial Guiding Principles

Financial guiding principles serve as a framework for getting the most satisfaction out of your money. They should influence the financial objectives you set, the money decisions you make daily, and how you approach your financial future. Here's a beginning list of principles to consider:

○ *Be an active manager of your money.* Effective financial management requires managing a budget and holding yourself accountable to your saving and spending priorities. If you don't keep your money on a leash, it will run away from home (and probably join the circus).

○ *Live below your means (or at least within your means).* Be frugal. Use the money you save to become more financially secure.

○ *Get the most satisfaction out of every dollar you spend.* Make the money you spend satisfaction-dense to enable your well-being. Ensure your money supports what you love the most (your ordered loves).

○ *Be a committed saver.* Strive to save at least 15% of your income for retirement. You may need to start at a smaller percentage, but then try to increase the rate yearly, especially if your income rises. If your employer offers a 401(k) retirement plan, participate in it and take advantage of the full company match (it's free money). What other future needs should you save for? Paying for college? Buying a home?

○ *Proactively manage financial risk.* Many experts suggest having an emergency fund available to cover at least six months of expenses (in case of a job loss or other hardships). If that's not possible today, strive to build to that over time. Another risk consideration is buying insurance to protect against loss and harm (life, health, auto, others).

○ *Minimize or eliminate debt.* Scrutinize all debt you take on and understand the terms and impact on your finances. Avoid credit card debt, if possible. If you're uncomfortable with your debt load, develop a plan to reduce it. That plan could include consolidating debt, increasing monthly payments (pay off higher-interest debt first), and leveraging debt relief or credit counseling experts for support.

○ *Be a wise investor.* When you invest, understand your objectives, investment options, and risk tolerance. That leads to the next item . . .

○ *Seek help.* You can leverage online resources or engage a certified financial expert for support.

○ *Give back.* Consider giving a portion of your income to those in need.

Which financial guiding principles resonate with you? Would you add any? As you identify your principles, you'll begin to get a sense of your financial objectives. You could have an objective to build a budget, develop a retirement savings plan, create a strategy to pay down debt, or establish an emergency fund. Your objectives will guide your financial plan. This is a nice segue to our next topic: leverage resources to build a financial plan.

## Leverage Resources to Build a Financial Plan

Financial planning can get complex, depending on your needs. A good financial plan could include: (1) quantified financial objectives, (2) a budget that reconciles your income and money allocations (living expenses, debt repayment, savings), (3) risk management considerations (emergency expenses, insurance), (4) investment and retirement planning, and (5) wealth management strategies (tax and estate planning). Your eyes may have glossed over after reading that list. But remember, a SAGe takes life step by step.

Let's assume you haven't played an active role in managing your money. Step one could be understanding what money you have coming in and where it's going, and then building a budget based on that information. That alone could be transformational. Building and managing a budget would empower your SAGe to make informed decisions about how to get the most out of your money to shape your financial well-being.

Once you have your budget working, you can focus on your next priority, whether that's building a retirement plan, creating a debt reduction strategy, or another objective. Take it step by step. And thankfully, there are plenty of resources to help you with each step.

A starting point can be leveraging online resources. You can access free and fee-based financial literacy courses and apps, blogs, calculators, and other tools through the internet. As an example, if you type "how to build a budget," "how much money do I need to retire," "budgeting apps," or "free financial course" into a search engine, you'll get a slew of resources.

You can also utilize financial experts. Many types are available—free and fee-based—including certified financial planners (CFPs), registered investment advisors (RIAs), robo-advisors (automated investment management services), financial coaches, brokers, accountants, and many others. You can access experts in person or online through banks and credit unions, financial services companies, pro bono groups and nonprofits, and community and government services. Research "find a financial advisor" online, and a world of possibilities will open up. Another approach to finding a financial expert is to get a referral from your trusted network.

Once you have identified qualified experts, performing due diligence is important to ensure you choose the right one. You'll want to understand each expert's credentials and experience level, how they partner with you, the services offered, and how they get paid (if at all). Another consideration is whether they have a fiduciary responsibility to put your interests above theirs. If they don't, they could recommend investments that pay higher commissions to them over options that would better serve your financial interests.

With the support of financial experts and resources, you can build a sensible financial plan that factors in your realities and guides you on a path to financial well-being. Once you have developed your plan, the next step is to actively manage your money so you stay on track with your plan.

## Be an Active Manager of Your Money

I'll share an excerpt from chapter 6 about adopting change that aligns with the essence of taking control of your money:

*As you make significant changes in your life, you will experience challenges. Everyone does. But what successful people do that separates them from the pack is they DON'T GIVE UP! They monitor their progress. They examine what's working and what's not, and adjust their approach accordingly. If they fall down, they stand up wiser from the experience. When they're successful, they celebrate. As they move forward, they bring their SAGe to the party and choose their best response to the reality that comes their way. By doing so, they may need to alter their plans or try different tactics. They may need to go back to the drawing board and reexamine their why, redefine what success looks like, or try other change adoption approaches. It's a part of the process. But their stick-to-it-iveness will lead to better results. It will bring satisfaction to their lives.*

To stay on course with your financial plan, it's important to engage with the state of your finances regularly. One of the best ways to do that is to leverage a budgeting app. There are easy-to-use apps that can help you build and manage a budget. Do you have money in the budget to go out to eat tonight? Are you on track with your savings objectives? The app will tell you that. Let the app do the heavy lifting to empower you to be an active money manager.

Other approaches that can help you stay on course include:

○ *Calendarize a monthly budget review.* After reconciling your budget each month (through an app or whatever works best for you), review how you did. Did you overspend in any budget category? Find out why. Do you need to reduce expenses next month to make up the ground? Then do so. Armed with insight into how you're doing, your SAGe can guide you in making adjustments as life happens.

○ *Leverage gamification features on budgeting apps.* Badges, progress bars, streaks, and challenges can motivate you to achieve your financial objectives. They also add fun to the mix.

○ *Proactively limit temptations.* To limit impulse purchases, you can opt out of marketing emails, avoid shopping malls or online marketplaces, shop with a list, and set spending limits on credit cards.

○ *Be intentional when you want to buy something.* Summon your SAGe, silence your Mischief Mind, and determine if the purchase is a need or a want. Does it align with your financial objectives? Does the purchase support an ordered love? Is there a better use for your money?

○ *Look for ways to reduce expenses to fund your financial security (pay down debt, build an emergency fund, save for retirement).* Use coupons, buy generic, buy in bulk, cancel subscriptions, eat out less, negotiate service rates, be energy efficient, carpool, wait for a sale before buying something, avoid impulse purchases—what else can you do?

○ *Leverage financial experts.* Besides partnering with you to build your financial plan, experts can help you monitor your performance and determine what adjustments should be made along the way.

○ *Utilize other change adoption techniques covered in chapter 6.* You can repeat affirmations about your ability to manage your money, set up a fun reward if you meet a financial objective, use visual management to keep your commitment to financial wellness in front of you, or get an accountability partner to serve as extra motivation to meet your financial intentions (a financial advisor could play that role)

As you become an active manager of your money, you'll increase your awareness about your spending habits and mindset toward money. Are there triggers that lure your Mischief Mind to waste money? Are there limiting beliefs about your ability to manage money? If so, work on shifting your mindset and changing your behaviors (utilize the practices you've learned in this book).

A theme throughout *The Wellness Ethic* has been to choose a love-centered response to your circumstances to promote well-being. Your SAGe always knows how to do that. But your SAGe is competing against your instant-gratification-loving Mischief Mind, especially when money is involved. Your Mischief Mind can throw a gorilla-sized monkey wrench into your financial intentions. It wants the largest house that the bank will approve. It covets a shiny, expensive car with all the latest features. It will only consider new family room furniture rather than buying a used set. Can you afford it? Your Mischief Mind is insulted you would even ask.

When you prioritize wellness, your SAGe puts the immature Mischief Mind in time-out. Your SAGe still wants gratification. But your SAGe understands that you want to be gratified throughout your life, which may require short-term sacrifices for longer-term gain. Life is full of trade-offs.

To choose your trade-offs wisely, consider the stress-reducing value of keeping life simple. Or the Stoics' counsel to detach from wants. Get to the heart of what is truly important in your life. That will help you prioritize what you do with your money; it will help you prioritize all aspects of your life.

When you keep financial wellness top of mind, leverage support, and manage a sound plan, you will improve your financial well-being. Step by step.

## Case Study—Small Changes Add Up to Big Changes

One of the most significant challenges in developing a financial plan and keeping to it is the trade-off between instant and future gratification. Take the example of Derek. Derek loves getting a premium cup of coffee at his favorite coffee shop before work each morning. The coffee costs $4. (Note: I prefer tea because it's what civilized people drink, but I'm not Derek—thank God.)

Each week, Derek's coffee indulgence adds up to $20. That may not seem like a big deal, but the financial impact is around $1,000 annually. If Derek had invested that amount each year for twenty years—instead of buying the coffee—and earned a 6% annual rate of return, it would have grown to be worth almost $40,000. That's a lot.

Should Derek make coffee at home (the cost is almost negligible), put it in a travel mug, and forgo his indulgence at the coffee shop? It may not provide the instant gratification he wanted, but it would help fund some of his longer-term financial objectives—$40,000 could go a long way.

## The Annoying Stuff

I'll just blurt it out: Lifestyle maintenance activities are annoying, time-sucking diversions from what I want to do—spend time with my family, write, practically anything but those activities! Yet they're required for my life to work. A messy house would make me unhappy. I must pay bills to keep receiving services. My car would develop an attitude if I didn't change its oil.

I'm my own worst enemy with lifestyle maintenance. One of my issues is I take on too many home improvement projects. And when I finish one, I get an idea for another. Then there's my devotion to my yard. Speaking of which, I must take a writing break to water sod that I put down to fix a patch of grass destroyed by a merciless army of machete-wielding chinch bugs!

I can't do everything that pops into my little brain. I need to focus on what's important. Whatever you engage in, you want it to be important to you—importance defined by *what you need*, such as making ends meet, being healthy, and pursuing experiences that fulfill you. When you engage in an activity, you also want it to make you happy. **When you do *important* activities that make you *happy*, you're operating in the sweet spot of your life.**

Since I don't like to disappoint my fans, I've developed a tool to sort through the relationship between *importance* and *happiness* in everything you do. The tool guides you on where you should focus your time and resources.

To fill it out, plot the activities you engage in according to their importance to you and the level of happiness you derive from them. Include lifestyle maintenance activities (cleaning, yard work, managing money, cooking, shopping, etc.) and other activities like work, exercise, hobbies, recreation, and so on. My example follows.

# Importance to You

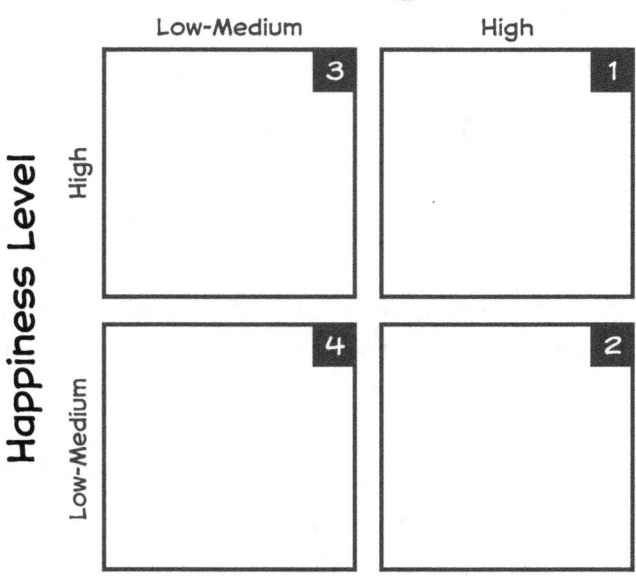

# Importance to Mark

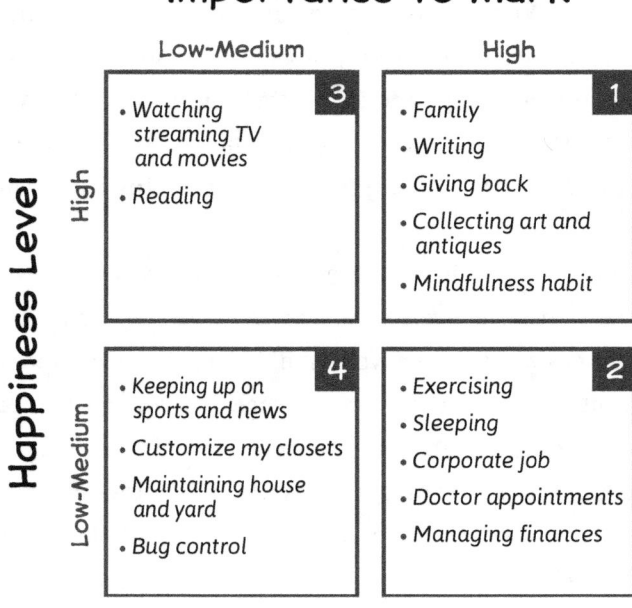

Here's some guidance on actions you can take based on the results:

○ *Quadrant 1 (High Importance/High Happiness)*: Immerse yourself in the activity—it likely aligns with your ordered loves or life purpose. My example: I need to free up more time to write.

○ *Quadrant 2 (High Importance/Low-Medium Happiness)*: Look for ways to boost happiness. My example: My corporate job is unsatisfying, and it takes up a lot of my time. I need to address that.

○ *Quadrant 3 (Low-Medium Importance/High Happiness)*: Engage in the activity but avoid overindulging or neglecting more important activities (strike a balance). My example: No changes needed.

○ *Quadrant 4 (Low-Medium Importance/Low-Medium Happiness)*: Consider dropping the activity as quickly as you would drop a radioactive potato engulfed in flames. Other options: spend less time on the activity, explore outsourcing, or find ways to make it more enjoyable. My example: The "customize my closets" potato was dropped with a resounding thud!

When you evaluate your Importance-Happiness chart, you'll likely reach three conclusions: There aren't enough hours in the day or money in your bank account to do everything you want to do, you don't always get as much satisfaction out of an activity as you could, and you sometimes engage in unimportant activities that don't bring joy.

Your time and resources are finite. That truth brings us back to the Thoreau quote I shared in chapter 11: "The cost of a thing is the amount of what I call life, which is required to be exchanged for it, immediately or in the long run." Everything you choose to do, including lifestyle maintenance activities, has an opportunity cost—you could have decided to do something else that might have been more satisfying.

Life is full of trade-offs. How can you make the right choices about what you do to boost satisfaction in your life? When feasible, a SAGe would respond to that challenge by:

○ finding creative ways to make activities more satisfying.

○ prioritizing the time and resources they allocate to activities that align with their life purpose and what they love, while spending less on everything else.

○ saying "no" to unimportant activities that don't bring them happiness.

○ accepting a lower standard of quality on unimportant activities if it saves time or money.

○ outsourcing activities that need to be done but are stubbornly dissatisfying.

By applying those principles to your lifestyle maintenance activities (and all other activities you engage in), you'll spend more of your precious time and resources realizing the meaning of your life—to feel and share love.

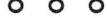

## Move Forward on Your Wellness Ethic Journey!

1. Detail actions you can take to make your lifestyle maintenance activities more satisfying (include change adoption strategies as appropriate).

```



```

2. Advanced Topics (going beyond the 80/20): If there are critical gaps in your financial literacy, develop a plan to close them. Additionally, explore approaches to decluttering your home and implement the ideas you like.

## Mark's Example

1. Detail actions you can take to make your lifestyle maintenance activities more satisfying (include change adoption strategies as appropriate).

*Small Action: Control my perfectionism by declining my next home improvement project—repainting my imperfect ceilings. By doing so, I'm saving two days of effort that will be allocated to writing my book.*

*Big Action: Outsourcing yard work will save a lot of time and hassle. I'll examine my budget to determine what's possible.*

# Design Your Life

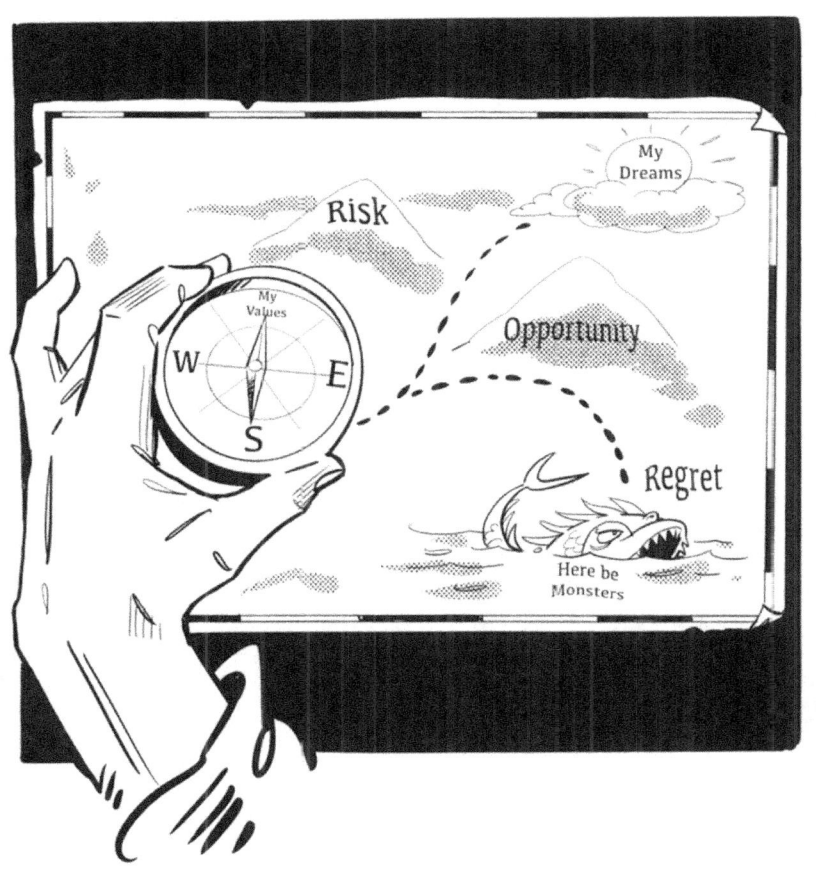

# CHAPTER 19

# A Story of Reinvention

I didn't see this one coming I should have—I had been begging the universe to deliver it for over a year.

Friday didn't start out as a consequential day. I had planned to work on a strategic initiative—my company had discovered a multimillion-dollar shortfall in its 2023 budget projections, and I was asked to help lead a program to find revenue opportunities to plug the hole.

The first item on my calendar was a 9:00 a.m. meeting with my manager. We connected each week to zip through project updates. This time, just as I started my briefing, he interrupted and told me our company was going through another round of layoffs. I wasn't surprised—layoffs were occurring throughout the tech sector—but I thought: *This is really stupid. I'll probably be asked to reduce my team. And my team is super-talented. I HATE layoffs!*

He then told me that *my job* was being eliminated. My last day would be in two weeks, and I would get three months of severance pay. The call ended quickly after that. When I hung up, I was at peace. It was as if my SAGe already knew how I would put this beanball into play.

I walked to my bedroom, where my wife, Kristen, was getting ready for the day, and told her the news. She was stunned—just months prior, she had been with me at a holiday dinner at my manager's house. But then she said something unexpected: *Now you'll be able to focus full-time on writing. That's what you've wanted.*

She was correct. I had been hoping for that. Desperately. Working my corporate job, while squeezing in twenty-plus hours of writing each week, was taking a heavy toll. Exhaustion oozed out of every pore in my body. It was like I was running through life on a 10% incline while wearing ankle weights. And I had been doing that for four years. No, make that thirty years when you consider all of my other side hustles.

From a professional standpoint, my book was what I was passionate about. But I knew I wasn't giving it the attention it needed to realize its full potential. I was all-in on my dream, but as a side hustle. That worried me. The book, in many respects, represented my life's work. I didn't want to shortchange it. I wanted to have two primary focuses: family and writing. The corporate job was a spare wheel. But I needed it to meet my financial obligations. Or did I?

How could I turn this layoff into a gift that would serve my life purpose? Could I focus my full-time efforts on writing and still make ends meet? I had done some financial planning in the past to see if it was possible, but I had decided not to leave my corporate job because I wasn't comfortable with the risk. But now that this opportunity was in front of me, what *really* was my risk tolerance? What did my SAGe think? Hmm.

Within five minutes of losing my job, my mind shifted into overdrive. If I were a full-time writer, I would devote all my energies to creating the best version of my book (as far as my talent could take it). I would immerse myself in the nuance of the writing craft, with every word and sentence carefully woven to tell the story I wanted to tell. Maybe my book would rise to the professional level and make a dent in the market; perhaps it wouldn't. But, man, it would be SO DAMN THRILLING to take the biggest professional dream I've ever had and go after it with no distractions, excuses, or regrets. Wow.

I needed this to happen. Writing *The Wellness Ethic* was my calling. The universe brought this opportunity to my door. There was a reason I was laid off, and it had nothing to do with the financial bind my company thought it was in. The universe was telling me it was time to pry open two dozen oysters; it was time to go all-in on my dream with my full-time energy and passion.

*How do I get to "yes"?* I pulled up our budget on my laptop. I projected how much money we would need to fund a two-year sabbatical from corporate America. I then focused on our revenue sources. When I added up our non-retirement savings, emergency fund, severance, and Kristen's expected salary if she reentered the workforce (she was willing to do that to help make my dream a reality), we could fund the sabbatical. This was getting interesting.

I thought more about it. What would I do if I had the gift of a two-year sabbatical? I could take a year to complete *The Wellness Ethic* and get it self-published. During that year, I could also get a health coaching certification (to supplement my life coaching credentials). Then, I would market my book and coaching services during the second year. If either pursuit gained traction, maybe I wouldn't need to return to corporate America. If they didn't, I would reenter the traditional workforce. I loved the plan! Two years to go after my dream with two potential revenue streams. But was it the best decision?

The essence of our decision came down to risk versus reward. The reward was by far the greatest for the two-year sabbatical. To have the opportunity to live my dream for at least two years was a once-in-a-lifetime opportunity. If it worked out, I would have a new career that I loved. It could be lucrative. If it fell short financially, I would still have experienced what would probably be the two most satisfying years of my life. And I would have a book on my bookshelf written by me and a legacy for my children. That would be fulfilling.

But what about the downside? If I took the sabbatical, I would face significant professional and financial risks. If I were out of the corporate game for two years and had to return, my skills would have fallen behind (AI is changing the landscape rapidly). That would impact the job level and pay I returned to.

From a financial standpoint, there would be two years that I wasn't earning or saving money (assuming, in the worst-case scenario, that my book or coaching didn't yield a meaningful return). That could push my targeted retirement age from sixty to my mid-sixties. Retiring by sixty has always been important to me.

Over the following week, as I considered what to do, I was contacted by a well-connected executive in my network who had heard about my layoff. He offered to champion my return to work by contacting people in his network. So now I had a promising path back to corporate America. If I pursued it right away, I could possibly find a job while still collecting severance (double pay!).

What an insane decision. Do I take the conservative path and immediately return to corporate America? If I returned, I would continue to write and still get my book self-published. It would just take years longer, and I may not be able to take it to the level I had hoped. There would also be a big *what-if* in my life if I didn't pursue my dream with my full-time energy. But life is full of trade-offs. I can live with that. I had accepted my reality when I turned down a film school scholarship two decades prior. I've never been a big risk-taker.

Or do I roll the dice and take the sabbatical? I was intrigued by what a full-time focus would do to my mastery of the writing craft. Would I discover that writing was what I was meant to do? Would it prove to be the difference-maker, in a game of inches, that propelled me to become a bestselling author? I had no idea. I can't control the future. But *what if*? I didn't want this *what-if* to turn into a *never-did*.

I then thought in Stoic terms. What is the realistic worst-case scenario, and can Kristen and I live with it? If the sabbatical didn't pan out financially, I would have to return to corporate America. But we would still have our retirement nest egg. Our house and cars were paid off, so we would still be debt-free. My daughters were out of college and independent, so they would be okay. I would have to work well into my sixties, but that would be tolerable. Kristen and I would still be together. The risks weren't really that bad—we would still have everything we *needed* to be happy, whether the outcome of the sabbatical paid off financially or not.

Still harboring some doubt, I looked to the Wellness Ethic Decision-Making model for more guidance. Taking the sabbatical aligned with my values. It would move me forward in an exciting direction. We could live with the risks. Kristen was fully supportive and viewed it as a win for both of us.

Then, my SAGe guided me to an old, trusted adviser to close the deal:

*I learned this, at least, by my experiment: that if one advances con-fidently in the direction of his dreams, and endeavors to live the life which he has imagined, he will meet with a success unexpected in common hours.*

—Henry David Thoreau

On February 28, 2023, with my wife's loving support and my trust in myself and the universe, I took the most significant professional risk of my career—I went all-in on becoming a full-time writer and life coach. Though I can't control how this decision will turn out financially, I know I won't have regrets. I'll be too busy nurturing the wonderful gift of my existence.

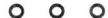

# Chapter 20

# Design Your Life as if Your Life Depends Upon It

You are now at a critical inflection point in your Wellness Ethic journey. You have been presented with insights, practices, and inspiration to help you thrive in an unpredictable world (where stupid things can happen). So, what do you want to do about it? **What do you need to do about it?**

Hopefully, you've already dabbled with lessons from *The Wellness Ethic* to create love in your life and the universe. If not, that's okay. What matters most is what you do moving forward. Do you choose to nurture the wonderful gift of your existence every day? When you do so, living a SAGe-inspired existence will become who you are. Your life will have a brilliant aura that will attract positive energy like fireflies attract wonder-struck children.

So, do you feel excited about moving forward? Are you motivated to seize the day? I have no doubt that you are! Let's celebrate this special moment by doing a workshop! What? That's not what you expected? I wanted to give you a free car, or at least a potted plant, to honor your commitment to well-being, but my accountant said the tax implications would be prohibitive. Sorry.

# Life Planning Workshop

There's no need to run for cover. The Life Planning Workshop isn't a big, foaming-at-the-mouth beast that will eat you for lunch, even though you may be nutrient-dense. We'll simply work through the change adoption process covered in chapter 6 (Why? – Define – Position – Do) to help you sort through how you want to move forward on your Wellness Ethic journey. You'll decide the pace and focus of your efforts.

You could take two months to build an exercise habit, and then focus next on healthy eating. After that, you could stack a mindful meditation habit on top of the habits you already formed. Or you may take on several focuses simultaneously. It's up to you. As you know, a realistic, well-thought-out approach is always preferred when introducing meaningful change into your life.

As a refresher, here's a summary of the Wellness Ethic foundation and pillars covered in this book. You can refer to it as we progress through the workshop.

| Wellness Ethic | 80/20 Components |
|---|---|
| Mind | o Nurture a positive mindset.<br>o Practice mindful engagement.<br>o Practice healthy detachment.<br>o Use emotional intelligence to regulate your happiness. |
| Body | o Science: Trust (but verify) the science related to your health.<br>o Treat: Implement preventive and reactive health approaches.<br>o Eat: Make healthy eating a habit.<br>o Exercise: Engage in regular mobility, cardiorespiratory, and strength exercises.<br>o Rest: Get consistent, restful sleep. |
| Spirit | o Embrace your life purpose.<br>o Love the universe of existence.<br>o Surrender to the ways of the universe.<br>o Have faith, if that's what you choose. |
| Relationships | o Utilize the LAST Relationship Model (Love, Accept, Share, Talk) to bring more love into your relationships. |
| Personal Pursuits | o Engage in satisfaction-dense personal pursuits. |
| Professional Pursuits | o Engage in satisfaction-dense professional pursuits. |
| Lifestyle Maintenance | o Move forward in the direction of financial wellness.<br>o Make the annoying stuff more satisfying. |

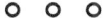

## Move Forward on Your Wellness Ethic Journey!

## **Why?** – Define – Position – Do

(1) Document why you want to focus on wellness. Get inspired as you think about the possibilities. Is your why a part of your spirituality? Does it define your SAGe? Does it enable your life purpose or align with the meaning of your life (to feel and share love)? Is it focused internally (be healthier, happier, more at peace) or focused externally (inspire others, support others, make the world a better place)? Or all of the above?

| Why I Am Committed to Wellness |
| --- |
|  |

## Why? – **Define** – Position – Do

(2) Define your wellness intentions for the next twelve months. Start by refreshing the baseline assessment you completed in chapter 2. Then, identify what you want to work on.

Current State: *Rate how you are doing with each Wellness Ethic component. Use a scale of 1 to 10, with 1 = "I'm performing abysmally" and 10 = "I'm thriving."*

Ideal State: *Rate where you would like to be in a year using the same scale as the Current State.*

Gap: *Gap = Current score minus Ideal score. If the gap is negative, there's room for improvement. Circle your top priorities.*

| Wellness Ethic | Current | Ideal | Gap |
|---|---|---|---|
| Love | | | |
| Mind | | | |
| Body | | | |
| Spirit | | | |
| Relationships | | | |
| Personal Pursuits | | | |
| Professional Pursuits | | | |
| Lifestyle Maintenance | | | |
| My Intentions for the Next Twelve Months | | | |
| | | | |

## Why? – Define – **Position** – Do

③ Develop a high-level plan capturing how you want to move forward with your wellness intentions over the next twelve months. Be careful not to overextend yourself by trying to do everything at once. In many cases, a sensible approach is to master a change or two, and then build upon that foundation by taking on the next challenge.

| Month | My Intentions | Change Adoption Approach |
|-------|---------------|--------------------------|
| 1 | | |
| 2 | | |
| 3 | | |
| 4 | | |
| 5 | | |
| 6 | | |
| 7 | | |
| 8 | | |
| 9 | | |
| 10 | | |
| 11 | | |
| 12 | | |

## Why? – Define – Position – **Do**

④ Document your thoughts on what will be critical to ensuring you realize your wellness intentions over the next twelve months (to the extent you can control). To assist you, here is a tool that covers the best practices from the "Do" phase in the change adoption process from chapter 6.

| Why | Define | Position | Do |
|-----|--------|----------|-----|

## Do

- ☐ DON'T GIVE UP!
- ☐ Monitor your progress.
- ☐ Choose your SAGe-inspired response to whatever happens.
- ☐ Adjust your approach based on what's working or not working.
- ☐ If you fall down, stand up wiser from the experience.
- ☐ Celebrate successes.
- ☐ Revisit the Why-Define-Position steps when necessary.
- ☐ Maintain a positive mindset.
- ☐ Understand that a transition is a process with ups and downs.

### Critical to My Success

To explore one-on-one life coaching services with Mark Reinisch or to access additional wellness resources, visit WellnessEthic.com.

# Mark's Example

## **Why?** – Define – Position – Do

(1) Document why you want to focus on wellness. Get inspired as you think about the possibilities.

| Why I Am Committed to Wellness |
|---|
| *By focusing on wellness, I will bring happiness and fulfillment into my life and share more love with my family, friends, and the world. It is the best way to nurture the wonderful gift of my existence!* |

## Why? – **Define** – Position – Do

② Define your wellness intentions for the next twelve months. Start by refreshing the baseline assessment you completed in chapter 2 (your scores may have shifted). Then, identify what you want to work on.

Date: June 2024

| Wellness Ethic | Current | Ideal | Gap |
|---|---|---|---|
| Love | 9 | 10 | -1 |
| Mind | 8 | 10 | (-2) |
| Body | 8 | 10 | (-2) |
| Spirit | 8 | 10 | (-2) |
| Relationships | 9 | 10 | -1 |
| Personal Pursuits | 8 | 8 | 0 |
| Professional Pursuits | 8 | 9 | -1 |
| Lifestyle Maintenance | 7 | 7 | 0 |

| My Intentions for the Next Twelve Months |
|---|
| Mind: introduce a daily meditation routine. |
| Body: lower weight by 15 pounds to help maintain healthy cholesterol levels. Experiment with intermittent fasting. |
| Spirit and Professional Pursuits: successfully transition to a full-time writer and life coach. This will serve my life purpose and help me get the most out of my professional pursuits. |

## Why? – Define – **Position** – Do

③ Develop a high-level plan capturing how you want to move forward with your wellness intentions over the next twelve months.

| Month | My Intentions | Change Adoption |
|---|---|---|
| Jul. '24 | - Pursue writing and life coaching (this is a focus each month). | |
| Aug. '24 | - Weight loss: 3 pounds | |
| Sep. '24 | - Weight loss: 3 pounds | |
| Oct. '24 | - Weight loss: 3 pounds | |
| Nov. '24 | - Weight loss: 3 pounds | |
| Dec. '24 | - Weight loss: 3 pounds | - Buy an antique after losing 15 pounds. |
| Jan. '25 | - Begin meditation routine (continue each month). | - Stack meditation habit with morning exercise routine. |
| Feb. '25 | | |
| Mar. '25 | - Try intermittent fasting; continue routine if I like the results. | - Align support of my wife. |
| Apr. '25 | | |
| May '25 | - Set new intentions for the next year. | |
| Jun. '25 | | |

## Why? – Define – Position – **Do**

④ Document your thoughts on what will be critical to ensuring you realize your wellness intentions over the next twelve months (to the extent
you can control).

| Critical to My Success |
|---|
| *The next twelve months will be quite dynamic. I'm well into year two of my sabbatical. I expect many ups and downs and pivots as life happens. Applying what I've learned throughout my Wellness Ethic journey—positive and growth mindset, choosing my SAGe-inspired response, the nature of transitions, applying change adoption tech-niques, etc.—will be essential. I feel very grateful to be able to go after this dream. It's what life is about!* |

# A Life Well Lived

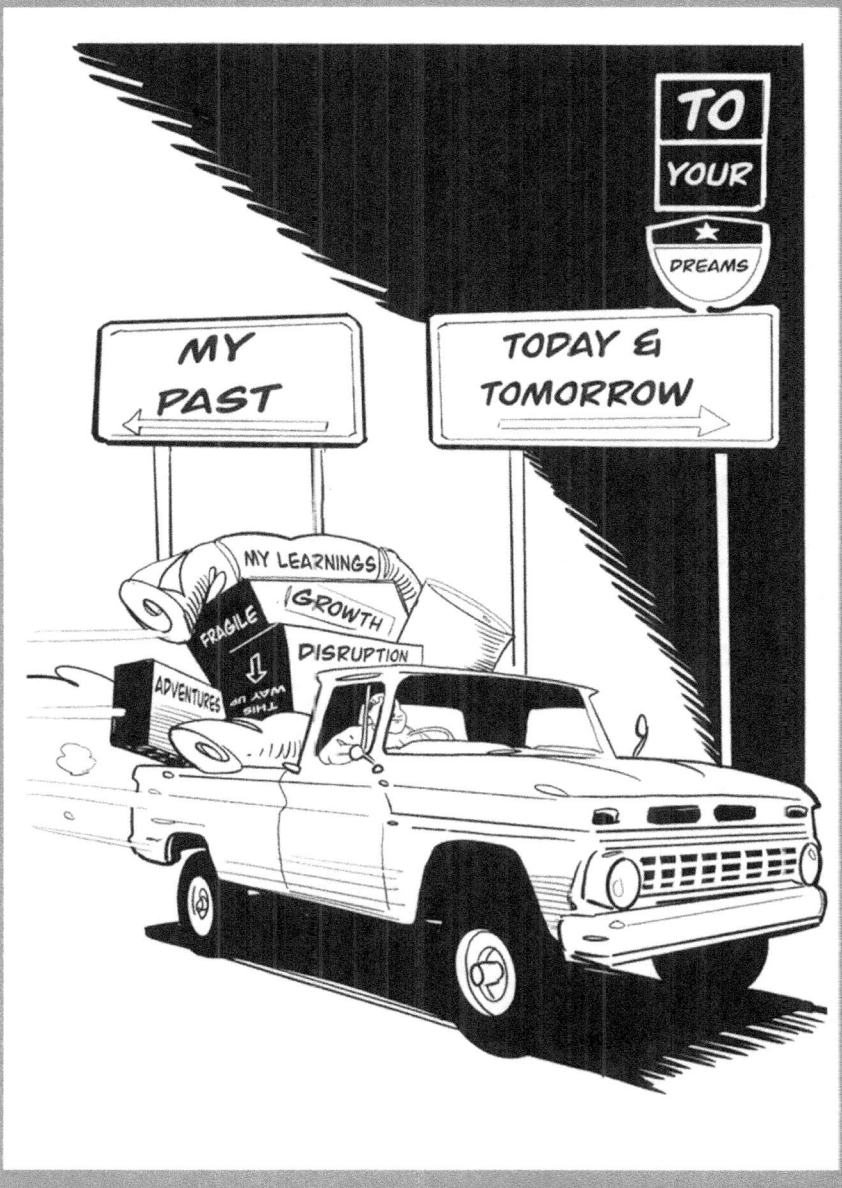

# CHAPTER 21

# A Story of Wisdom

You *can* go home again. It will certainly be different. You'll be different. But a significant part of you that was there is with you now. Your past molded your character, beliefs, and passions. It memorializes your growth and the love you've created in the universe. What can you learn from your past to serve you now and in the future?

That's what I want to explore before I close out this book. I'm fifty-four as I write this. I've lived more years than I have remaining, which is quite humbling. In previous chapters, I examined much of my post-college life through the Wellness Ethic lens, but I haven't popped open the lid on my formative years. I know how to take care of that.

## It's Road Trip Time!

I was born in Albany, New York, and lived in Upstate New York for the first thirty years of my life. To complete my road trip, I'll travel north from my home in Charleston, South Carolina, to Albany, then head farther north toward the Canadian border. During that journey, I'll tour all the places I lived during my K-12 school years—Berne, Ticonderoga, Queensbury, and Beekmantown—and will complete my trip by visiting my college alma mater, Rensselaer Polytechnic Institute (RPI), in Troy, New York.

For each stop, I'll design satisfaction-dense experiences that channel my younger self and transport me back in time. But I'll also allow myself to go with the flow and see where that takes me. I can't wait to see what I learn from this experience. This should be fun.

After a nine-hundred-mile drive, my first stop was Berne, which is thirty minutes outside of Albany.

## Berne, NY (ages 4 to 7)

I didn't have high expectations for my visit to Berne. I only lived there a couple of years and hadn't been back in close to fifty. I planned to drive by my former house, and that would be it. Satisfaction density would be limited by design.

As I drove past my old home on a Saturday morning, it was anticlimactic—I saw a house that I vaguely remembered. What I was most interested in was the farmhouse next door. My brother and I were friends with the children who had lived there. It was a vast property with a pond, streams, barns, rolling fields, and farm animals—a perfect setting for children to disavow their comfort zones and fearlessly explore, especially in the age of free-range parenting.

I slowed down as I reached the farmhouse. I saw a field that I had played in. It was there that I hit my first baseball, rode horses, and even shot flaming arrows—made out of cattails—at my dear friends (long story).

I then saw an elderly lady on the property, weeding her front yard. Could that be Rachel? Rachel was my friends' mother, and I adored her back then. Today, she would be in her eighties. *Do I stop and talk to her? But I'm not 100% sure that's her. Even if it is, she won't remember me after fifty years. Besides, I'm an introvert. I don't do things like that.* I drove on.

My daughters' voices barged into my head and scolded me: *Go back, Dad! You're gonna regret not finding out if it was Rachel! And we thought the whole purpose of this road trip was to create memorable experiences!?* I knew I had to get out of my comfort zone and return. *Ugh.* I turned my car around.

I pulled up in her driveway and rolled down my window. The lady approached, holding a garden hoe. I told her who I was, and her face lit up with delight. It was Rachel! She remembered me!

I exited my car and had a wonderful twenty-minute conversation about our families and my memories of playing at her house. She couldn't stop laughing when she reenacted the story of when I was in her home, thunder shook the house, and she raised her arms in jest as she told me she was the "Goddess of Thunder!" Five-year-old Mark proceeded to cry hysterically as he ran back home to the safety of his mother! I was amazed that she still remembered that story fifty years later. Her vitality at her age was remarkable. You could tell she had found ways to maintain her zest for life over the years.

After that twenty-minute visit, I could have driven back to Charleston and viewed my road trip as a success. That's how moving my experience was. I was honored that she remembered me and I had left an impression that stayed with her throughout her life. I was also inspired by seeing a lady in her eighties who got up early in the morning to maintain her sprawling farm.

**Throughout my life, I have never once regretted summoning the courage to get out of my comfort zone.** It has defined my growth and made my life interesting. I need to do that more often.

## Ticonderoga, NY (ages 7 to 8)

For this leg of my trip, I wanted to add exercise to my experience (satisfaction density!), so I walked two miles from my hotel to my old house.

When I got there, I reconnected with the joy I felt as an eight-year-old when the new baseball cards were released for the season. I would walk alone to a country store a mile away to buy them. I would then sit for hours in my bedroom, in awe of my heroes, as I opened packs and read the stats on the backs of the cards. That began my lifelong passion for collecting things.

When I left the neighborhood, I stopped at a cemetery across the street and explored. I walked past hundreds of tombstones spanning centuries.

It moved me that each grave represented a lifetime of dreams, adventure, happiness, and disappointment. Their lives had flown by in a flash, and now they rest in peace.

I then thought that, if I'm fortunate, I might have thirty to forty years left before joining them (*knock, knock, knock*). I'm not trying to be morbid. It just speaks to the nature of our earthly existence—it's brief by design. That's why it's important to intentionally manifest as much love as you can every day of your life.

I toured historical sites throughout the rest of the morning— Ticonderoga has a rich Revolutionary War and War of 1812 heritage—and was in my element. But the most memorable part of my Ticonderoga visit was almost an afterthought. I always had wanted to visit an antiques shop in a historic town. Maybe they would have an inventory of historical relics from their region.

So I dropped by Lonergan's Antiques, which is housed in a creaky old barn that is an antique in itself. What an inventory! The highlight was dozens of cannonballs and rifles from the Revolutionary War through the Civil War. I purchased a Revolutionary War bar shot (a cannon projectile that looks like a barbell) and couldn't wait to add it to my home collection.

Though the antique shop was impressive, the most delightful part of the visit was an engaging chat I had with the shop owner, a gentleman in his seventies. His passion for history was infectious. By owning an antiques shop and sharing history with others, he was doing what he was created to do.

The Ticonderoga visit deepened my conviction that **I must spend every precious day of my brief time on this planet living my life on purpose and surrounding myself with what I love.**

## Queensbury, NY (ages 8 to 11)

I attended school at Queensbury from second through fifth grade, so my memories were more vivid than at my previous stops. I wanted to reconnect with those times and had the perfect satisfaction-dense experience in mind.

Back then, my friends and I would ride our bikes five miles from our neighborhood to Aviation Mall. It was always a detour-filled adventure that allowed me to explore my independence. For my return visit, forty-plus years later, I planned to park my car at the mall, walk to my house, soak up memories along the way, including seeing my old elementary school, and then head back.

To put myself in the right frame of mind, I created a playlist of my favorite songs from that era, including classics like "Boogie Wonderland," "Y.M.C.A.," "Shake Your Groove Thing," "Le Freak," and "Born to Be Alive." I was excited about this leg of my journey and looked forward to listening to disco music, exercising, and feeling the emotions of my youth.

I started my walk, and within thirty minutes, I saw a ten-year-old kid riding his bike in a parking lot. That could have been me over forty years ago! My mind traveled back to those times, and it felt real. I wanted to ask the kid if I could take his bike for a spin to improve the satisfaction density of my experience, but I didn't think he'd understand. Nor would the authorities.

I continued to walk and was really getting into the music. As I listened to "Y.M.C.A.," I had a brilliant thought that was Einstein-level genius: I should do the Y.M.C.A. dance moves to fully connect with the moment. *But I'm walking on a busy road; I would look funny. Mark! Your SAGe doesn't give a damn about your whiny excuses! Find a way to "yes!"* I knew I had to do it.

The trick was to respect the moves but to do them discreetly. So I did them in a way that a casual observer would think I was just stretching my arms as I walked. But I knew better, which amused the hell out of me. Here's a re-creation, in my Charleston neighborhood, of my Y.M.C.A. buffoonery:

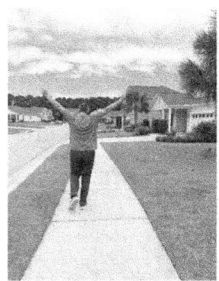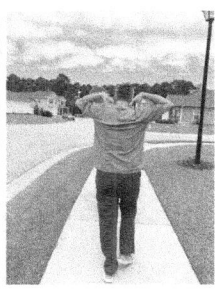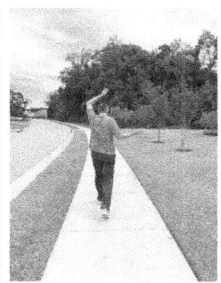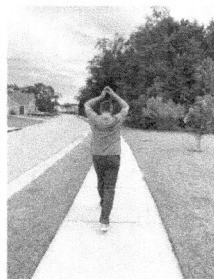

The journey to my house generated fond memories of friends, girlfriends, Little League Baseball, shenanigans in class, and carefree summers. I was brought back to an uncomplicated time filled with exploration and wonder. **I need to be more carefree and recapture the joyful discovery of my youth.**

## Beekmantown, NY (ages 12 to 18)

Beekmantown followed the same playbook as Queensbury—do a lot of walking, connect with memories, and, of course, create a killer playlist. My Beekmantown soundtrack was dominated by 1980s alternative bands like R.E.M., The Cure, Depeche Mode, Oingo Boingo, The Church, and Love and Rockets.

I started at Beekmantown school. I parked my car, put in my earbuds, hit play on Spotify, and headed toward my house a mile away.

When I got to my road, hardly anything looked familiar. I had traveled that road over a thousand times—walking to school, meeting up with friends all hours of the day and night—but it was like a foreign land. In the twenty-five years since I had last visited my neighborhood, there seemed to be twice as many houses. I even walked a hundred feet past my old house before realizing it!

I was taken aback by how much had changed—houses, landscapes, and people I knew who had moved away. I found myself yearning for the way things used to be. But then I caught myself and realized that change is constant. I wouldn't want to be the exact person I was twenty-five years ago—why would I want other people or places to stand still?

I had formed my identity at Beekmantown—my character, humanity, and passion for creativity. This is where I had come of age, where I learned to be a leader rather than a follower. Everything that I had become could be traced back to these roots, and that foundation steadied me as I branched out in my life. That is also what happened to everything in my old neighborhood. It had leveraged the foundation of its roots to grow and evolve. The change I saw fascinated me when I viewed it like that. I embraced it and thought about how perfectly it represented the ways of the universe.

**Change is a curious phenomenon that keeps life engaging and full of intriguing growth opportunities *if we embrace it*.**

## RPI—Troy, NY (ages 18 to 23)

My primary reason for visiting my alma mater was to see if they had named a building after me. They hadn't. That was disappointing. But it taught me a valuable lesson: **If you want a building named after you at a college, you'll need to donate more than $50 to the institution over your lifetime.**

## Summing Up My Road Trip

My road trip was one of the most enjoyable experiences of my life. It was a perfect blend of adventure, nostalgia, history, music, exercise, and catching up with old friends and family. The satisfaction density was off the charts.

I left with the prevailing belief that the reward of life revolves around people and the love and experiences you share. I had crafted this road trip to revisit the places that shaped who I am today. Seeing old houses and neighborhoods was neat, but connecting with my friend Gary in Beekmantown (and videoconferencing with his mother), my friends Sean and Margaret in Rochester (I took a detour to see them), Rachel in Berne, my relatives in Albany, and the antiques shop owner in Ticonderoga were the highlights of the trip.

I also left the road trip convinced I shouldn't leave my house without adult supervision. The number of turns I missed while driving was incalculable. I got lost walking on the small RPI campus, and it's basically a straight line of buildings. I searched for my room key in my hotel room for nearly an hour, only to realize it was still in the door lock. I drove to a local bakery in Maryland that was ten minutes away, got epically lost, and ended up eating breakfast at a Dunkin' Donuts an hour later. And I had a GPS. Why am I like this?

But even my misadventures were part of the adventure. The road trip helped me reconnect with my formative years and put my life in perspective. I'll share that perspective with you now.

## My Life in Perspective

When I thought about the totality of my life, I kept returning to Irish playwright George Bernard Shaw's quote: "Life isn't about finding yourself. Life is about creating yourself." How did I create myself? Since I have to be me, I created a diagram to help me wrap my arms around my life journey:

# A Bird's Eye View of Mark's Life

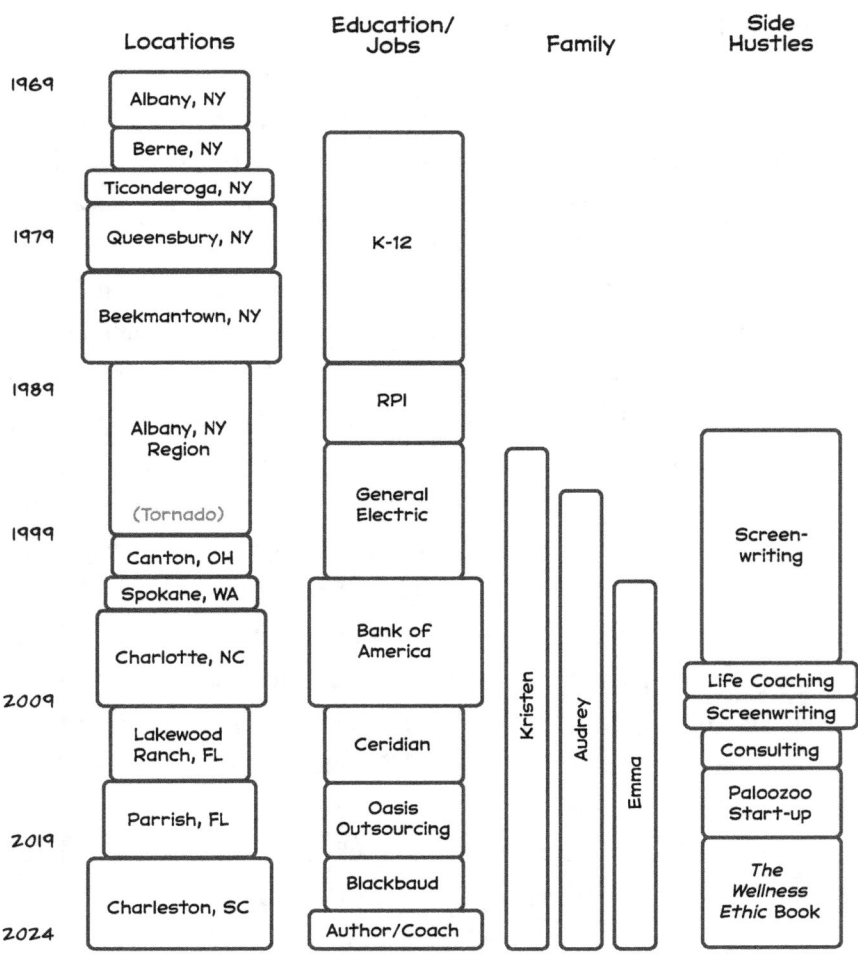

As I look at the chart, I find it fascinating how little I knew about what was in store for me once I graduated from RPI. There was no way I could have foreseen the countless adventures that would unfold as I crisscrossed the United States and lived in so many diverse places. Who could have predicted a wicked tornado would level my cherished home in Mechanicville? That my professional life would include working for Fortune 500 companies and midsize firms in diverse industries, and during that career, I would weather the storm of four layoffs? That I would have a loving family, and they would prove to be the most fulfilling part of my life? That I would passionately pursue side hustles to manifest my dreams? My life journey boggles my mind, just like your life journey probably boggles your mind.

I've experienced so much change throughout the years and so much growth. Every box in my diagram represents my humble attempt to nurture the wonderful gift of my existence. The boxes represent relationships, adventures, successes, and challenges. They represent love.

My life has been perfectly imperfect. Many people have achieved more financial success and professional accolades than me. Many people have better aligned their lives to their life purpose. And they may be happier and more fulfilled than I am. But I'm not living their life—I'm living mine.

I've done my best to make love and character central to my life. I've been challenged with stupid stuff, but who hasn't? It's a part of everyone's journey. Obstacles lead to opportunity, engagement, and growth. They're an indispensable ingredient to a fulfilling life.

My life is the perfect life of an imperfect husband, father, son, brother, friend, writer, creator, leader, collector, entrepreneur, life coach, humorist, and servant. I'm thrilled with that. It's a good life.

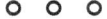

# CHAPTER 22

# Advance Confidently in the Direction of Your Dreams

We've come a long way in this book. We've come a long way in our lives. This crazy little thing called life is awe-inspiring. So much opportunity. So much joy. A fair share of stupid stuff that we can't control. But often, the challenges engage us and bring out our best. Through trials, we develop wisdom and sharpen our capabilities—it's how we grow. And when we taste success or partake in the pleasures of life, our happiness runs deeper because we know what it's like to want but not to have.

We understand that the good and the stupid are fundamentals of how the unpredictable universe operates, and we surrender to that reality. We nurture the wonderful gift of our existence every day because we know that's why we were put on this planet. With that noble purpose, we live the meaning of our life, to feel and share love. It's what inspires our devotion to wellness. It's how we define our success, which we measure in units of love. Love is core to how our Self-Actualized Genius accepts, frames, and responds to what happens in our life.

We're about to conclude our time together. We've shared ideas and inspiration about wellness. But really, this book is about life possibilities. Focusing on wellness is the best method to get the most out of those possibilities.

The secret to thriving in this universe is to move forward in your life with a love-centered purpose focused on the components of wellness—mind, body, spirit, relationships, personal and professional pursuits, and lifestyle maintenance—that bring you the most satisfaction and make the world a better place. Your happiness and fulfillment soar when you stay focused on what you can control—your mindset and loving responses to what happens in your life—not outcomes outside your sphere of influence.

None of this will ever be "perfect," especially your wellness. You would be utterly foolish if you expected it to be. It's not the way of the universe. But that's why the Wellness Ethic exists: to help us thrive in an unpredictable world (where stupid things can happen).

A constant theme of this book has been to keep it simple by focusing on the vital few breakthrough ideas, the 80/20 concepts that will benefit you the most. So here's my take on the five most important concepts to live your life with a Wellness Ethic (it's the 80/20 of the 80/20!).

○ *Live a spiritual life.* Embrace your life purpose. Love the universe of existence. Surrender to the ways of the universe. Have faith, if that's what you choose. Living a spiritual life puts you in the best position to realize the meaning of your life, to feel and share love.

○ *Serve your body.* To promote health, apply the STEER model (Science, Treat, Eat, Exercise, and Rest). You can fully engage in life when you're as healthy as possible (to the extent you can control).

○ *Surround yourself with those who bring love into your life.* Wellness is dependent upon thriving relationships. Spend quality time with the important people in your life. Get out and mingle with the community. Make new friends. Distance yourself from toxic people. Make cultivating loving relationships a top priority.

○ *Seek satisfaction-dense experiences.* Pry open the oyster and get the most out of your personal and professional pursuits. Align them with your life purpose and what you love. Don't settle for blah; eliminate never-dids.

○ *Boost your happiness by empowering your SAGe to accept, frame, and respond to your circumstances.* By doing so, you'll stay aligned with your life purpose and values. You'll cultivate a healthy mindset. You'll adopt meaningful change. You'll choose the most loving response to what happens in your life. You'll put yourself in the best position to thrive.

That's how you nurture the wonderful gift of your existence. As for me, I've been living those values for over five years as a part of my Wellness Ethic experiment. I've had a lot of trials to test how the concepts work. I wouldn't characterize it as trial and error. I view it as trial and success. Every step forward has yielded progress. I've either had positive outcomes—some have been transformational—or I've fallen short but have been armed with insights to try again. To give you a sense of what my Wellness Ethic journey has done for me so far, I'll share a few outcomes:

○ *I wrote this book!* It took six years of crazy hard work and sacrifice, but now I feel like I have a grasp on what life is about, and I have a legacy for my children. That's very satisfying.

○ *I have made significant strides with everyday happiness.* I've made it a regular practice to mindfully engage in the wonder around me. I am more intentional with how I spend my time by seeking satisfaction-dense experiences. I'm about 75% where I need to be with surrendering to what I can't control, detaching from the toxicity of current events, and silencing negative self-talk. That's good progress, and I'll keep working on it.

○ *I am more fulfilled with my life.* I feel like I'm living it on purpose. I am more grateful for my blessings, especially my relationships. I no longer compare myself to others. I've forgiven myself for past mistakes. I feel like what I've accomplished in my imperfect life reflects my essence, and I'm good with that.

○ *I have finally lowered my cholesterol to an acceptable level without taking medication!*

○ *My growth put me in a position to confidently take the biggest risk in my professional life.* My life satisfaction took off after I left corporate America to pursue a writing and coaching career.

Hopefully, you have experienced positive results with the stuff you've put into practice. But whatever you've done, wherever you are, you're on a journey. **You're on a never-ending quest to connect with the beautiful love inside of you and to feel it and share it with the world every day of your glorious life.** Your Self-Actualized Genius will guide you on your journey, so you're in good hands.

Nurture the wonderful gift of your existence, my friend, and advance confidently in the direction of your dreams!

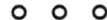

# Odds & Ends

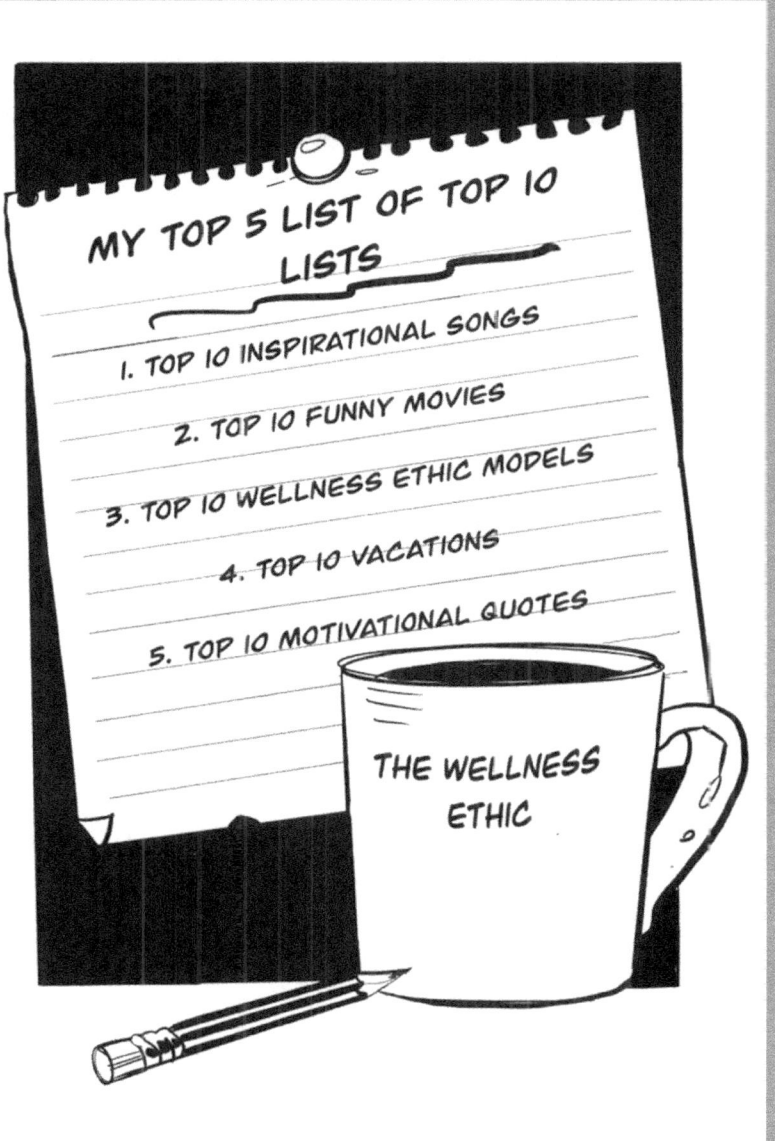

# Self-Indulgent Top 10 Lists

You may wonder why I included top 10 lists in my wellness book. There are a few reasons. First, I thought it would be helpful to offer lists of books, music, movies, and other topics that could inspire you on your Wellness Ethic journey. Second, I wanted to encourage you to have fun and engage in a creative activity like creating your own top 10 lists.

But really, the main reason is that I look for excuses to indulge myself with things I enjoy, and I love creating lists. I also revel in the intoxicating feeling of righteousness I get when I judge the work of others to determine the "best of the best." But I probably shouldn't mention that—it's not very spiritual. I'll have to remember to delete that admission prior to publication.

## Top 10 Songs That Instantly Put Me in a Good Mood

1. "Day Is Done"—Peter, Paul and Mary
2. "Marie"—Leon Redbone
3. "Take Five"—The Dave Brubeck Quartet
4. "Guantanamera"—Pete Seeger
5. "Bye Bye Bill Bailey"—Pete Fountain
6. "I'll Remember April"—The Modern Jazz Quartet
7. "Livin' Thing"—Electric Light Orchestra
8. "Twist"—Tones on Tail
9. "A Day in the Life"—The Beatles
10. "Just Like Heaven"—The Cure

## Top 10 Biographies That Inspire Me

1. *Alexander Hamilton*—Ron Chernow
2. *Robert Kennedy and His Times*—Arthur M. Schlesinger, Jr.
3. *Steve Jobs*—Walter Isaacson
4. *John Adams*—David McCullough
5. *Unbroken: A World War II Story of Survival, Resilience, and Redemption*—Laura Hillenbrand
6. *A Man Called Intrepid*—William Stevenson
7. *Team of Rivals: The Political Genius of Abraham Lincoln*—Doris Kearns Goodwin
8. *The Last Lion: Winston Spencer Churchill*—William Manchester
9. *A Promised Land*—Barack Obama
10. *Leonardo: The Artist and the Man*—Serge Bramly

## Top 10 Books That Improved My Life (Modern)

1. *Man's Search for Meaning*—Viktor Frankl
2. *Change Your Thoughts—Change Your Life*—Dr. Wayne W. Dyer
3. *Solve for Happy*—Mo Gawdat
4. *Transitions*—William Bridges
5. *Working with Emotional Intelligence*—Daniel Goleman
6. *The Success Principles*—Jack Canfield
7. *The 7 Habits of Highly Effective People*—Stephen R. Covey
8. *The Seven Principles for Making Marriage Work*—John M. Gottman, Ph.D.
9. *The Blue Zones of Happiness*—Dan Buettner
10. *The Purpose Driven Life*—Rick Warren

## Top 10 Movies—Laugh-Out-Loud Comedies

1. *This Is Spinal Tap*
2. *A Fish Called Wanda*
3. *Raising Arizona*
4. *The Naked Gun*
5. *The Jerk*
6. *Airplane!*
7. *Bridesmaids*
8. *Superbad*
9. *There's Something About Mary*
10. *Monty Python and the Holy Grail*

## Top 10 Favorite Musical Albums—All Genres

1. *Abbey Road*—The Beatles
2. *Carreras Domingo Pavarotti in Concert*—José Carreras, Plácido Domingo, Luciano Pavarotti
3. *Les Misérables*—10th Anniversary Concert at London's Royal Albert Hall
4. *Graceland*—Paul Simon
5. *What's Going On*—Marvin Gaye
6. *Decade*—Neil Young
7. *Live 1966: "The Royal Albert Hall Concert"*—Bob Dylan
8. *The Joshua Tree*—U2
9. *Collaboration*—The Modern Jazz Quartet with Laurindo Almeida
10. *The Sun Years*—Johnny Cash

## Top 10 Battle Bots That I Desperately Wish Existed

1. Scaredy Bot
2. Jell-O Mold Bot
3. Atomic Detonator That Also Throws Grenades Bot
4. Fragile Glass Bot
5. Ding Bot
6. Invisible Cloak Bot
7. Wet Recycled Cardboard Bot
8. Out-of-Order Bot
9. Balloon Animal Bot
10. Tater Bot

## Top 10 Remaining Items on My Bucket List

1. Get in the ballpark of becoming a Self-Actualized Genius.
2. Make ends meet through self-employment.
3. Learn how to paint and develop a level of proficiency.
4. Reconnect with as many friends from my past as possible.
5. Publish book #2.
6. Fully fund a college education for someone I don't know.
7. Have meaningful experiences in as many countries as possible.
8. Produce an independent film of one of my screenplays.
9. Transition to an organic, plant-based diet.
10. Read the sacred texts of the world's major religions.

# Let's Promote Wellness in the Universe!

If you have enjoyed *The Wellness Ethic* and believe it can benefit others, you can spread the word in many ways. *The Wellness Ethic* is self-published and self-marketed, so I appreciate your support! Here are some ideas to help promote wellness in the universe:

- Leave a favorable review of *The Wellness Ethic* wherever you purchased the book and in other forums.

- Create a social media post about *The Wellness Ethic* to inspire people to move forward on their wellness journey.

- Buy *The Wellness Ethic* for your friends and family members.

- Start a Wellness Ethic club and meet regularly to support and celebrate the positive things people do to move forward in their lives.

- Be a wellness beacon by *leading with love* in all that you do. You will bring joy to yourself and others. Love is all upside!

Thank you for engaging with *The Wellness Ethic*!

With gratitude,

*Mark*

Mark Reinisch

# Acknowledgments

It can take a village to educate an idiot like me, which was the case when I wrote *The Wellness Ethic*. Many people played an essential role in helping to make this book a reality. I am forever grateful for their considerable expertise, feedback, encouragement, and generosity!

- Editors: Stuart Horwitz, Nancy Pile, Emma Reinisch

- Illustrator: Danny Burgess

- Expert Reviewers: Dave Albertson, Dolores Calicchio, Shane Doll, Aida Hitti-Zeidan, James Morrison, Monica Mutter, Dr. Andrea Walter, Dr. Sarah Weinsztok

- Beta Readers: Mary Jo Anderson, Ryan Eckenrode, Sean Kavanagh, Kristin King, Lee Layton, Carolyn Parker, Audrey Reinisch, Kristen Reinisch, Lauren Reinisch, Robert Reinisch, Laura Dela Rosa, Erik Seversen, Chris Singh, Kate Tant

- Publishing Support: 1106 Design

- Proofreaders: Julie Ann Ehrenzweig, Ellen Tarlin, 1106 Design

- Painting in Chapter 10: *Still Life with Claude Lorrain Landscape* by Sherrie Wolf (www.sherriewolfstudio.com)

- "About the Author" Crater Lake Photo: Blake Shaffer

**It was a joy and an honor to partner with so many talented people!**

# Endnotes

## Background Stuff

1   A.H. Maslow, "A Theory of Human Motivation." *Psychological Review* 50, no. 4 (1943): 370–396, https://doi.org/10.1037/h0054346.

## 2. For the Love of Wellness Models

1   Wayne W. Dyer, *Change Your Thoughts—Change Your Life: Living the Wisdom of the Tao* (New York: Hay House, 2013).

## 4. Respond Perfectly to the Imperfect

1   Viktor E. Frankl, *Man's Search for Meaning* (Boston: Beacon Press, 1959, 1962, 1984, 1992, 2006).

## 6. Jack of No Change, Master of None

1   W. Wood and D. T. Neal, "A New Look at Habits and the Habit-goal Interface," *Psychological Review* 114, no. 4 (2007): 843–863, https://doi.org/10.1037/0033-295x.114.4.843.
2   Charles Duhigg, *The Power of Habit: Why We Do What We Do in Life and Business.* (New York: Random House, 2012).
3   K. Teo et al., "Prevalence of a Healthy Lifestyle among Individuals with Cardiovascular Disease in High-, Middle- and Low-Income Countries," *JAMA* 309, no. 15 (April 17, 2013): 1613–1631, https://doi.org/10.1001/jama.2013.3519.
4   William Bridges and Susan Bridges, *Managing Transitions* (New York: Hachette Go, 2009).

## 8. You Don't Need a Chatbot to Discover the Meaning of Life

1   David Brooks, *The Road to Character* (New York: Random House, 2016).

## 10. Calm Psyche, Happy Lifey

1 Sonja Lyubomirsky, Kennon Sheldon, and David Schkade, "Pursuing Happiness: The Architecture of Sustainable Change," *Review of General Psychology* 9, no. 2 (2005): 111–131, https://doi.org/10.1037/1089-2680.9.2.111.

2 Laura Sapranaviciute-Zabazlajeva et al., "Link between Healthy Lifestyle and Psychological Well-Being in Lithuanian Adults Aged 45–72: A Cross-Sectional Study," *BMJ Open* 7, no. 4 (April 1, 2017): e014240, https://doi.org/10.1136/bmjopen-2016-014240; Pauline Hautekiet et al., "A Healthy Lifestyle Is Positively Associated with Mental Health and Well-being and Core Markers in Ageing," *BMC Medicine* 20, no. 1 (September 29, 2022): 328, https://doi.org/10.1186/s12916-022-02524-9.

3 Elaine Mead, "6 Benefits of Happiness According to the Research," PositivePsychology.com, June 5, 2019, https://positivepsychology.com/benefits-of-happiness/.

4 Carol S Dweck, *Mindset: The New Psychology of Success* (New York: Ballantine Books, 2006).

5 David D. Burns, *Feeling Good: The New Mood Therapy* (New York: William Morrow, 1980).

6 Mihaly Csikszentmihalyi, *Flow: The Psychology of Optimal Experience* (New York: Harper and Row, 1990).

7 Daniel Goleman, *Emotional Intelligence* (New York: Bantam Books, 2006).

## 12. Healthy Living Tastes Great and Is More Fulfilling

1 Carl Zimmer, "How Many Cells Are in Your Body?" *National Geographic*, May 3, 2021, https://www.nationalgeographic.com/science/article/how-many-cells-are-in-your-body.

2 Yanping Li et al., "Impact of Healthy Lifestyle Factors on Life Expectancies in the US Population," *Circulation* 138, no. 4 (July 24, 2018): 345–355, https://doi.org/10.1161/circulationaha.117.032047.

3 "Centers for Disease Control and Prevention," Centers for Disease Control and Prevention, https://www.cdc.gov/alcohol/about-alcohol-use/moderate-alcohol-use.html.

4 Jennifer Lubell, "Diet Patterns That Can Boost Longevity, Cut Chronic Disease," American Medical Association, February 16, 2023, https://www.ama-assn.org/delivering-care/public-health/diet-patterns-can-boost-longevity-cut-chronic-disease.

5 Amby Burfoot, "Two Major Studies Just Showed What a Processed Diet Can Do to Our Bodies," Science Alert, June 27, 2019, https://www.sciencealert.com/there-s-now-research-to-back-the-trend-of-scorn-towards-processed-food.

6 Walter J. Crinnion, "Organic Foods Contain Higher Levels of Certain Nutrients, Lower Levels of Pesticides, and May Provide Health Benefits for the Consumer," *Alternative Medicine Review: A Journal of Clinical Therapeutic* 15, no. 1 (2010): 4–12, https://pubmed.ncbi.nlm.nih.gov/20359265/#:~:text=However%2C%20 reviews%20o f%20multiple%20studies%20show%20th; Catherine Roberts, "Stop Eating Pesticides," *Consumer Reports*, August 27, 2020, https://www.consumerreports.org/health/food-contaminants/stop-eating-pesticides -a1094738355/#:~:text=But%20many%20 ex-perts%20remain%20concerned.

7 "What Is MyPlate?" USDA, 2020, https://www.myplate.gov/eat-healthy/what -is-myplate.

8 Edwin McDonald, "Eating Slower May Help with Weight Loss," *U Chicago Medicine*, November 28, 2018, www.uchicagomedicine.org/forefront/weight -management-articles/eating-slower-may-help-with-weight-loss.

9 C. D. Reimers, G. Knapp, and A. K. Reimers, "Does Physical Activity Increase Life Expectancy? A Review of the Literature," *Journal of Aging Research* 2012, no. 243958 (2012): 1–9, www.ncbi.nlm.nih.gov/pmc/articles/PMC3395243958.

10 Sammi R. Chekroud et al., "Association between Physical Exercise and Mental Health in 1.2 Million Individuals in the USA between 2011 and 2015: A Cross-Sectional Study," *The Lancet Psychiatry* 5, no. 9 (September 2018): 739–746, doi:10.1016/S2215-0366(18)30227-X.

11 Cleveland Clinic, "From Head to Toe: The Benefits of a Cardio Workout." Cleveland Clinic, May 8, 2023, health.clevelandclinic.org/the-many -benefits-of-a-cardio-workout.

12 "Physical Activity Guidelines for Americans," Health.gov, health.gov/our-work/ nutrition-physical-activity/physical-activity-guidelines.

13 Amanda E. Paluch et al., "Steps per Day and All-Cause Mortality in Middle-Aged Adults in the Coronary Artery Risk Development in Young Adults Study," *JAMA Network Open* 4, no. 9 (September 3, 2021): e212.24516.

14 Haruki Momma et al., "Muscle-Strengthening Activities Are Associated with Lower Risk and Mortality in Major Non-Communicable Diseases: A Systematic Review and Meta-Analysis of Cohort Studies," *British Journal of Sports Medicine* 56, no. 13 (January 2022): 755105061.

15 Jay Summer, Dr. Abhinav Singh, "Eight Health Benefits of Sleep,' Sleep Foundation, February 29, 2024, www.sleepfoundation.org/how-sleep-works /benefits-of-sleep.

## 14. Are You Super-Connected?

1 Robert Waldinger, "What Makes a Good Life? Lessons from the Longest Study on Happiness," TED Talks, November 2015, video, 12:38, https://www.ted.

com/talks/ rob-ert_waldinger_what_makes_a_good_life_lessons_from_the _longest_study_on_ happiness?language=en.

2    John Mordechai Gottman and Nan Silver, *The Seven Principles for Making Marriage Work: A Practical Guide from the Country's Foremost Relationship Expert* (New York: Harmony Books, 2015).

# About The Author

**M**ark Reinisch is an author, life coach, and entrepreneur specializing in personal transformation. He has decades of executive experience in corporate America, having driven transformation programs to help people and companies realize their vast potential. As side hustles, he founded a social media start-up, shepherded it to a successful buyout, and has written a dozen comedic screenplays. His dry wit comes along for the ride in all that he does.

Mark resides in Charleston, South Carolina, with his wife and herd of cats. He loves going on adventures with his two adult daughters. You can visit Mark at WellnessEthic.com to access his wellness blog and life coaching services.

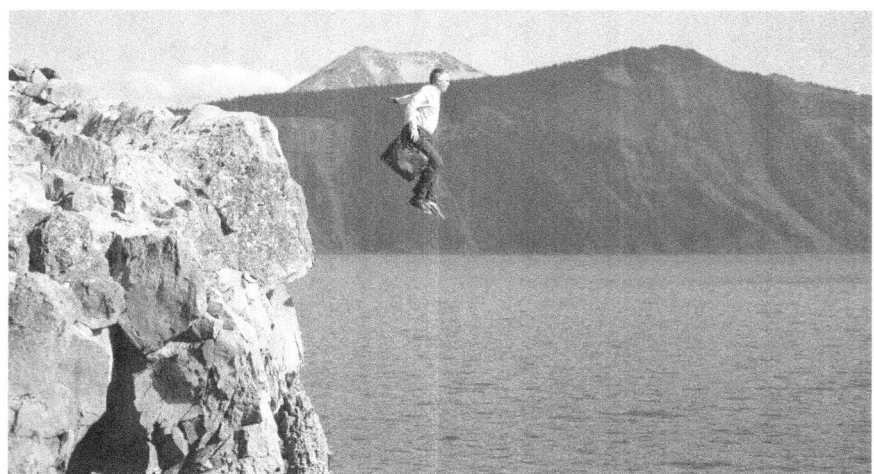

The cliff-diving photo was taken on August 26, 2023, at Crater Lake, Oregon. Yes, that's Mark jumping thirty-five feet into the frigid water in business attire. And, no, it wasn't photoshopped. It's the real deal.

Four years prior, he visited Crater Lake with his daughter Emma. She jumped in at that spot, but he didn't. He's afraid of heights and never understood why a person with brain cells would choose to swim in freezing water.

He regretted not taking the plunge, so he jumped in years later when he returned to the national park. It represented his progress on his Wellness Ethic journey—he overcomes fear in pursuit of satisfaction-dense experiences. And by wearing business attire, it was symbolic of taking a leap of faith and leaving corporate America to pursue a career as a writer and life coach.

# Remember

*Your life journey has no destination. Banish that limiting belief.*
*You don't need to arrive anywhere because you're already there.*

*Don't let disorienting fog obscure your vision of a purposeful life.*
*When you stay true to your inspiring purpose, you realize*
*your life's meaning, to feel and share love.*

*Embrace your past, but don't live in it. The wisdom and grace learned*
*from the mistakes and triumphs of yesteryear will serve a better today.*

*Dream about the future, but don't be beholden to the precision*
*of your dreams. You live a fulfilled life by experiencing the*
*spiritual essence of why you were born into this world,*
*not by achieving an outcome beyond your control.*

*Engage in the precious now and nurture the wonderful gift*
*of your existence every moment of your life. Your loving*
*responses to life's happenings and your positive mindset*
*in the moment will determine your happiness.*

*Be kind to your one-of-a-kind self, always.*